TAMING THE BLACK DOG

Winston Churchill was no stranger to depression. It was he who called it the Black Dog and in so doing gave the affliction a recognisable identity.

Until *Taming the Black Dog* was published in August 2004 there existed no definitive self-help programme for sufferers, or their relations, friends, and colleagues. Following approbation by leading professionals in the field, as well as by readers, this book has been reprinted.

Taming The Black Dog is the foundation of residential courses for service men and women embarking on civilian life including those suffering from Post Traumatic Stress Disorder.
www.remount.net

"I have reviewed many books of relative merits but never have I reviewed one which I recommend everyone to read, that is until I read Taming the Black Dog *… It talks about depression in everyday language … It never talks down to you … It deals with the psychological and physical elements. It is a practical and comprehensive handbook for surviving depression … It is a really helpful book."*
Professor Stuart Kotze holds professorships in Behavioural Psychology at Oxford, Aston and Warwick Universities

"This brave and honest book is a dispatch from the front line of depression. Patrick Ellverton deals with the relationship of depression and alcohol consumption head on. Two chapters which I specially recommend are firstly 'Your Emotions' in which he tackles a notoriously difficult subject with startling lucidity. The second is 'Helping a Friend' which also deals with the relationship between doctor and patient."
Robert Beaumont of the Charlie Waller Memorial Trust which funds research by GPs into the treatment of depression

"Compelling reading."
Amelie Mustapha of Depression Alliance, the leading UK charity for people with depression

TAMING THE BLACK DOG

PATRICK ELLVERTON

howto**books**

To my grandchildren James and Holly

Published by How To Books Ltd
Spring Hill House, Spring Hill Road, Begbroke, Oxford OX5 1RX
Tel: (01865) 375794. Fax: (01865) 379162
info@howtobooks.co.uk
www.howtobooks.co.uk

The right of Patrick Ellverton to be indentified as the author of this work has
been asserted by him in accordance with the Copyright, Designs and Patents
Act 1988.

First edition 2004
Reprinted 2005, 2007, 2008 and 2009

British Library Cataloguing in Publication Data
A catalogue record for this book is available from the British Library

ISBN 978 1 85703 999 3

Produced for How To Books by Deer Park Productions, Tavistock
Cover design by Baseline Arts Ltd, Oxford
Illustrations by David Mostyn
Typeset by Baseline Arts Ltd, Oxford
Printed and bound by Cromwell Press Group, Trowbridge, Wiltshire

NOTE: The material contained in this book is set out in good faith for
general guidance and no liability can be accepted for loss or expense incurred
as a result of relying in particular circumstances on statements made in this
book. The laws and regulations are complex and liable to change, and readers
should check the current position with the relevant authorities before making
personal arrangements.

Contents

Acknowledgements

To Amelia Mustapha of Depression Alliance who gave me the encouragement to proceed in the early days and Suzi Rogol, the editor of *Good Time* magazine, who published the first chapter as an article.

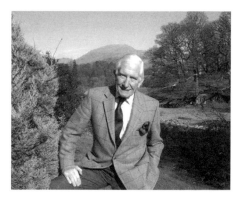

To Giles Lewis my publisher and Nikki Read the commissioning editor who decided to give me a run, and to Francesca Mitchell my editor for her clarity of thought and suggestions. Also David Mostyn my illustrator for so successfully giving the Black Dog an image for everyone to visualise.

Specially to Susie Storey for her lively and constant interest, without whose practical help the book might never have found a publisher.

'Who are you?' I was asked. I replied, 'I am me the same me as ever was but I am also a little part of everyone against whom I have brushed throughout my life.'

So this book is also dedicated to all of you too numerous to recall.

Patrick Ellverton

Then turn again to your task. Look forward, do not look backward. Gather afresh in heart and spirit all the energies of your being, bend anew together for a supreme effort. The times are harsh, the need is dire, the agony seems infinite but the power of commitment and perseverance hurled united into the conflict will be irresistible.

Adapted from a speech by **Winston Churchill**, 1915

Depression – a definition

Almost everyone experiences depression at some time in his or her life. Depression is more than just a debilitating feeling – it is a profound psychological and physical experience, which affects the body's whole physiology.

Depression can be actually painful and it is dangerous. If you are seriously considering suicide as a solution to your depression, please get help NOW. Call your doctor at once for immediate clinical help, or telephone one of the crisis lines listed in Appendix 2 of this book, provided by Samaritans, SANE, or Depression Alliance.

Depression is often defined as a condition in which a number of specific symptoms persist for at least one month. If you have four of the following symptoms you are probably depressed. If you have five or more you are definitely depressed.

1. Feelings of worthlessness, self reproach.
2. Inappropriate guilt.
3. Recurrent thoughts of suicide.
4. Weariness and loss of energy and feelings.
5. Diminished ability to think and concentrate.
6. Loss of interest or pleasure in usual activities.
7. Decrease in sexual drive.
8. Continuing state of worry and apprehension.
9. Insomnia or hypersomnia.
10. Poor appetite with weight loss or increased appetite with weight gain.
11. Physical inactivity or hyper-activity.

Along with these symptoms, the body's physical functions can become unbalanced as well. Constipation and changes in the menstrual cycle are common and you may feel cold, weak and sluggish.

Depression may occur as a brief, transient event or it may be a lifelong struggle, as with the author of this book.

When depression results from the death of a loved one, the end of a relationship or the loss of a job, the feelings may be appropriate and normal. Indeed a period of grief and sadness is essential. Treatment is generally not needed unless the depression is severe enough to make someone non-functional and entertain suicidal thoughts.

However, the general rule is that people with depression should seek a medical evaluation. Symptoms that look like depression might be caused instead by a specific medical condition, such as a thyroid complaint, hormonal imbalances or a side effect of medication. The involvement of a medical practitioner is not just sensible; it is very reassuring and will help to reduce the level of anxiety in both the sufferer and their loved ones.

The prime rule is to consult your doctor, particularly if you think that you might be suffering from manic depression. Your doctor will be able to advise you on the professional help that is available to you. Then this book will help you get back on your feet again – permanently.

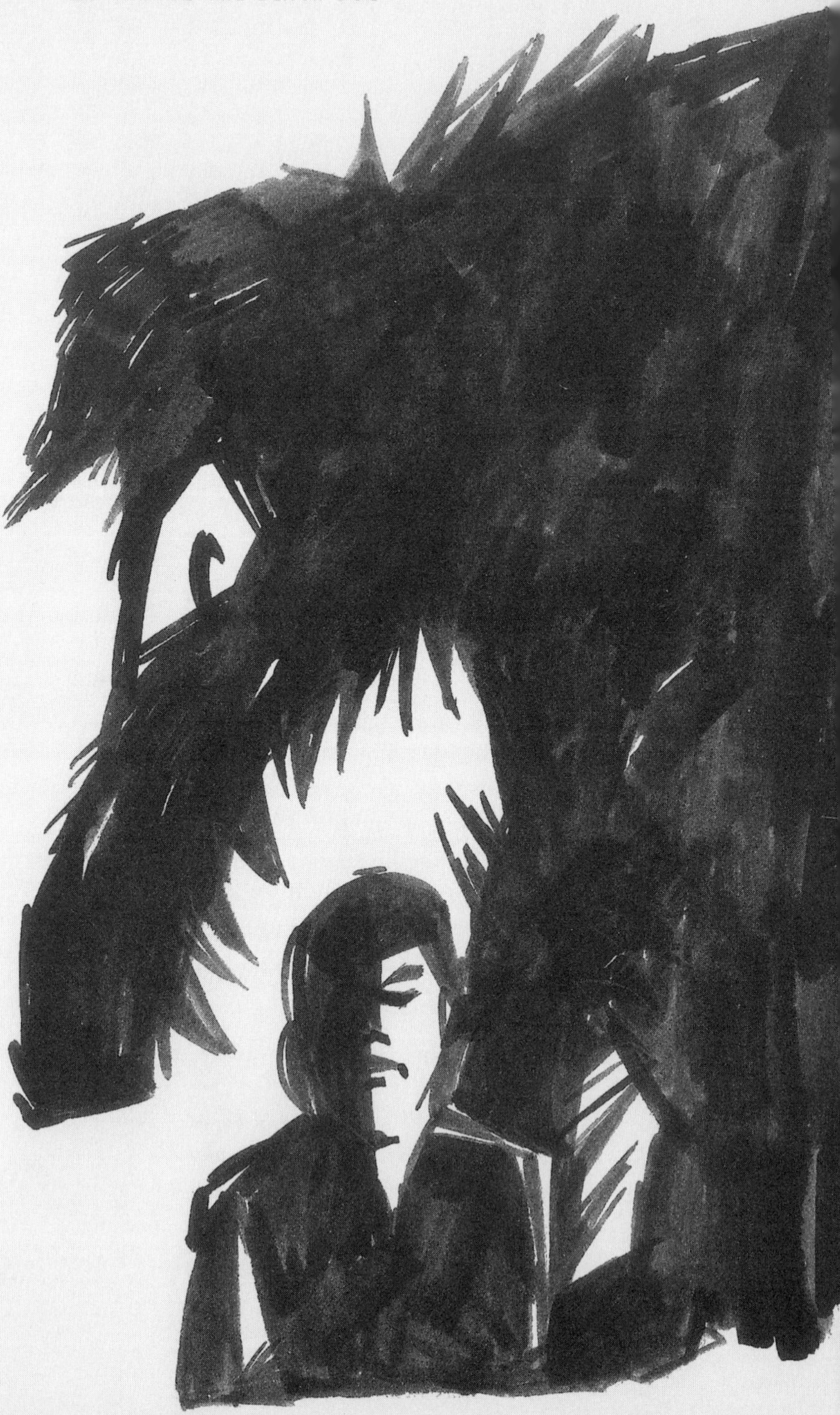

Chapter 1
Introduction

A GREY, OPPRESSIVE CLOUD HANGS OVER EVERYTHING it seems, from horizon to horizon. It diminishes light and neutralises the colours around us. It inhibits love, spoils enjoyment, denies humour, magnifies legitimate worries and results in a sense of purposelessness. It is a mental affliction, which we call depression. Fortunately for most sufferers it is not continuous and comes in bouts. Winston Churchill gave it an identity and called it the Black Dog.

The sooner depressives can give their affliction an identity, the easier it is for them to deal with it. The Black Dog is not just a mental affliction. It is a creature, which stalks our brains and undermines bodily functions. But it can be tamed practically and decisively. How can I be so sure? I have done it.

I had fought and wrestled with the beastly thing throughout my life, from being a schoolboy, then a tank officer, merchant banker and television director. It seemed that for most of my life I had suffered from an ever-present weariness.

I had no alternative but to share the family view that I was simply lazy and needed to pull my socks up, as my father would often say. The result was that despite my achievements, I had low self-esteem, which was camouflaged from my friends and colleagues by an outgoing, apparently cheerful and entertaining personality. Nobody, but nobody, at that time would have believed that I was suffering from depression, and the concept of low self-esteem was unknown to most people then. Certainly it was not a subject for healthy young people to bother contemplating.

Low self-esteem is arguably the most destructive aspect of clinical depression because it is not obvious, yet it inhibits and even stops the development of love and understanding in the intimate relationships of marriage and parenthood. The Bible tells us to 'love thy neighbour as thyself'. If you do not love yourself, it's hard lines on your neighbour, and particularly your spouse and children – and, yes, your parents!

It caused me to view the setbacks in my life as monumental failures and lead me to move to something new in order to escape from what I perceived as ignominy in that role.

Winston Churchill was helped, no doubt, by the adrenalin-pumping environment of politics, but in the hiatus preceding a speech would sink into a depression and would resort to the whisky or port decanter. I too, unwittingly, was using alcohol as a medication to overcome the lack of confidence in my ability to be socially amusing. Without alcohol I thought that I lacked what Noel Coward called 'a talent to amuse' – something that we all need in one form or another if we are to feed our relationships with warmth and fun.

This was the start of my being alcohol-dependant, which in time contributed to the breakdown of both my marriages and family life and unquestionably handicapped my career. It blunted the incisive cutting edge of my ability.

If this is ringing a bell – whether or not you use alcohol in this way – then read on, because it is the substance of my concern with depression. My reason for writing this book is to share with you the methods I adopted to tame the Black Dog and for us to look together towards the blue skies for ourselves and for those we love.

THE NATURE OF THE BEAST

Depression is like a demonic threatening beast and if it is to be tamed, we need to understand its nature and when it prowls. A doctor, like a veterinary surgeon sedating an animal, uses drugs to ameliorate the behaviour. However, the process of healing the wounds that the Black Dog has already inflicted must be carried out by the victims themselves. The good news is that we really can do this ourselves and benefit immeasurably in so doing.

What are these wounds? They are the bad mental habits which have developed during the time we have been afflicted. Negative thinking, lack of purpose, a feeling of futility affecting everything we embark on, and worst of all – fear. Fear of the future. Fear of being unable to cope with the everyday tasks of life. Fear of failure in our projects and even fear of success. Fear, like almost all the components of depression, is a natural emotion, which has jumped out of its life-saving box and is neutralising the dynamics of life enjoyed by a healthy person, such as love, friendship, adventure, creativity, sport and simply enjoying the richness the world has to offer.

The result of all this is low self-esteem, which undermines all our relationships and endeavours. Over the years these negative propensities become established habits, which we need to eradicate in our journey to the blue skies.

Fortunately, fear that is divorced from imminent danger is an attitude of mind and can be put back where it belongs by positive thinking and by consciously challenging it head on. Grasping the bull by the horns is the principle.

HOLDING THE WRONG HAND

Remember the adage that success is born out of mind over matter and so is failure. That is why depression is so debilitating. It undermines physical well-being and health, because depressives may eventually tend to capitulate to the unremitting agony and seek relief in short-term alleviation.

They use alcohol to alleviate their anguish and provide transitory cheerfulness, after which they suffer even deeper depression. They resort to comfort eating, and sometimes become seriously overweight. The distraction of television also gives temporary respite and like alcohol allows the brain to escape from its life-stimulating functions. Indeed, the combination of uncritical television-watching and alcohol is the most demotivating poison around and has resulted in the birth of the most unhealthy of depressives – the self-induced couch potato. (*See chapter* 15.)

The physical results of unchecked depressiveness can include obesity, high blood pressure, sexual impotence, diabetes, arthritis, utter despair and suicide. But the good news is that you can extricate yourself from this downward spiral.

Medication will stabilise a sufferer long enough for you to put together a new act, but this you need to do yourself. Psychological counselling, in my opinion, is needed by only a very small number of sufferers and if inappropriately administered can be counterproductive. I believe that the counselling of a trusted friend with a similar spectrum of interests is more likely to be beneficial.

> *The thrust of this book is to steer you away from introspective studies of the nature and effects of your depression and to focus your mind on squeezing it out by thinking positively and living creatively.*

The process of replacing the bad physical and thinking habits with good ones is therapeutic in itself, and confidence, morale and self-esteem all begin to re-establish themselves rapidly. The associated sense of achievement is a tremendous motivator in accelerating the process.

That is the nature of the beast, which we have to tame and then manage. Yes, I'm afraid that those of us who have an inherited propensity for depression will spend the rest of our lives keeping the Black Dog in his kennel. But the good news is that the actions I am recommending, irrespective of whether you are a temporary sufferer or like myself have inherited the beast, can enhance everyone's enjoyment of life beyond recognition.

WHAT CAUSES DEPRESSION?

Depression for most people is caused by the impact of exceptional circumstances on their lives and may eventually disappear altogether. However, the mental damage will still need repairing.

Post-natal depression and menopausal depression are the most common among women. It is recognised that men, too, can suffer depression seriously in mid-life and, because they keep it to themselves, suffer deeply. The cause is connected with the change in hormones at these times possibly associated, particularly in the case of men, with a recognition of the transitory nature of life and concern about the purpose of their existence.

The trauma of an accident or bereavement can result in depression. Indeed, inadequate grieving for a loved one often has a long-term depressive effect.

Failures in professional life can have a devastating effect on some people, knocking their confidence, damaging their ego, neutralising their sex drive and destroying their self-esteem.

Debt and money worries are common causes of depression throughout society and are seriously corrosive to relationships and self-esteem.

Irrespective of which category is relevant, the method of recovery is the same and the techniques can be utilised on a continuing basis to enhance the enjoyment of life, long after the Black Dog has been kicked into touch.

So now to horse, let's gallop on to the blue skies.

SOME PROCEDURES FOR TAMING THE BLACK DOG – IN BRIEF

- **Purchase a page-a-day diary.** Record in it the times and circumstances of each Black Dog attack during the day and night and make a note about what you were or were not doing at the time.

- **The most immediate mood-lifter is exercise.** Walk briskly for 40 minutes every morning and use the exercise programme in Chapter 17, or jog for 20 minutes whenever you can. If you are overweight and have not taken exercise for some time, start with the exercises and a 15-minute walk each day for the first two weeks, then increase to 30 minutes for the next two weeks, before moving up to 40 minutes. If you are under medication, consult your doctor. Outdoor exercise is a key element in recovery.

- **Go out of your way to do something for someone else each day** – a helping hand for an acquaintance or neighbour, a loving gesture for your spouse, an unexpected present for your children. It need not cost money but must involve your time, effort and devotion.

- **Look for the best in others** and say something congratulatory to someone every day of your life.

- **Plan and minimise alcohol consumption.** When socialising be sensible and decide beforehand how many glasses you are going to allow yourself over what time. When you've reached your planned limit, leave. Driving will reinforce the necessity to be careful.

- **Eat nourishing food and carefully plan your eating regime.** Cut out all junk food, avoid sandwiches and reduce carbohydrates like potatoes, bread and other starches. Eat a preponderance of fruit and vegetables each day, with meat and high energy food at just one meal. Go for a walk afterwards.

- There are one or two highly reputable international companies who provide naturally resourced meal replacement programmes which are excellent in achieving **high energy-to-weight ratio levels.** People who are seriously overweight should consider one of these. The best programmes are supervised and are supported by a panel of doctors and nutritionists. One advises the US Olympic athletics council on nourishment. Proper nourishment is as important to the depressive as it is to the athlete because energy is needed in taming the Black Dog – and, by the same token, so is fitness.

- **Take up a sporting activity** like walking, cycling, tennis, golf, water sports, riding, gliding, sailing, football, badminton. Something with a personal achievement goal. Spectator sports do not count and have little value for the purpose of defeating the Black Dog. Like alcohol (with which they are often associated) and television, they are simply ephemeral distractions. Depression cannot exist when the adrenaline is surging. Try bungee jumping.

Learn to pray or meditate

Every morning and evening set on one side five minutes to pray. Surprised by this? Don't be. Praying is the most powerful healing process.

Praying is simple. Talk to God about your concerns and ask him for inspiration and guidance in taming the Black Dog. Understand that He comprehends everything, so when you talk to him there is no point in being anything but completely honest with him, and most importantly with yourself.

The Bible and the Koran teach that God is love and love is the greatest positive influence in calming the wayward emotions, which constitute depression.

As well as – or instead of – prayer, meditation is an extremely helpful and effective way of taking a break from our anxieties and miseries and finding deep relaxation, tranquillity and renewed energy.

Start and end the day right

If you have a partner, when you get up each morning and when you go to bed each night, say 'I love you'. If you have children, tell them that you love them. When you see yourself in the mirror, say, 'I love you. We are having a rough time but you are doing well. We're winning. I'm proud of you and I love you.'

That last person is the most important one today.

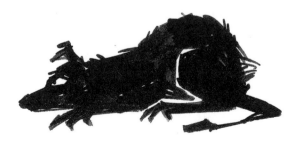

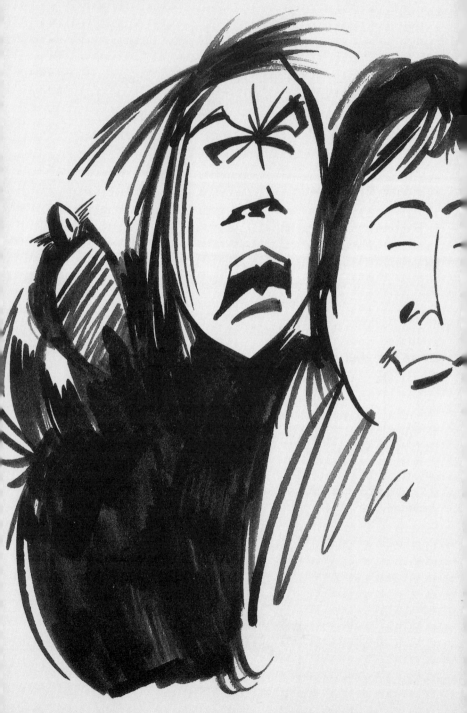

Chapter 2
Your emotions

WE HUMAN BEINGS HAVE A SOPHISTICATED EMOTIONAL SYSTEM, which equips us to handle every situation we encounter. We see it working in other people every day and we experience it operating in ourselves.

It permits us to love and to fall in love. It allows us to appreciate beauty and to enjoy our world. It warns us of impending danger. It equips us to handle day-to-day crises and to compensate for the calamity of losing a limb or becoming blind or having to live on our own. It is a terrific survival kit. However, its effectiveness depends on maintaining a balance between the negative emotions and positive ones.

We are like a sailing ship, which has to sail through good weather and bad weather – through seas which are sometimes rough and sometimes calm. We have to keep ourselves in balance by trimming our sails to the wind, sometimes steering a more comfortable course, securing shifting cargo, and in threatening times discarding some of it.

In the case of us humans we accumulate unwanted baggage as we proceed through life. From time to time we have to rid ourselves of some of this baggage when assailed by the threatening squalls of a depression. Our emotional system becomes unbalanced and we keel over unnaturally towards the negative side of our makeup, and then in the case of manic depressives swing back uncontrollably and keel over dangerously towards the positive side. As with sailing ships this oscillation is dangerous and will increase in magnitude if it is not brought under control.

BRINGING YOUR EMOTIONS INTO BALANCE

When this happens to us, we have to rebalance our system. This is a recurring theme in this book: getting ourselves balanced.

To help grasp how a normal emotion, when out of control, can undermine the balance of our minds, let us consider the emotion of fear for a moment. Fear, when out of its box, is the most debilitating and wayward emotion. It will stop us in our tracks. It will actually physically paralyse us, prevent us from doing the things that we know we could and should be doing. It is possibly the first emotion to become irrational when we suffer from depression.

Yet normally fear is a vital element in our survival kit. It cautions us to be careful. It makes us consider alternative ways of achieving an objective. It triggers the release of adrenaline and equips us to fight or flee from an impending threat. When properly managed it actually facilitates our progress towards our goals and in this respect takes on a positive aspect. Let it get out of control and it will paralyse our initiative and create hopelessness.

All our emotions are like this and need to be kept in balance. That's what I'm asking you to grasp – the concept of balance. To overcome depression we must first of all identify which of our emotions are out of balance and what underlying causes are contributing to the imbalance.

MUSIC AND YOUR EMOTIONS

Music can be a great help in taming the Black Dog, particularly when you are alone. After exercise, it is the greatest mood lifter if you access it properly. Every kind of music can have its place on a lonely day – swing, show music, jazz, classical both old and contemporary, rock, pop. Music is a natural component of every human being's consciousness. It is there to be appreciated like a beautiful view and is a natural associate of memories. More than that it can be a mental stimulant, which is beckoning us to enjoy and understand it. Like tasting good wine the more you become accustomed to listening to it the greater will be your appreciation and the more rewarding its effect.

When I am by myself I have music playing all the time. It accompanies my writing, thinking, household chores and gardening. There are a number of radio programmes which provide music all day and there are very good concerts in the evening. They all provide a foundation for a music collection. Listening to music is infinitely more beneficial than mindlessly watching TV.

Playing a musical instrument will invariably dismiss the Black Dog from your presence. If you played an instrument in the past but let it drop years ago, try taking it up again. Don't mess about, go to a music shop and buy or order a definitive music tutorial for your chosen instrument and devote 30 minutes each day to learning it afresh. You will find that it is tremendously rewarding and you can always pick it up when the Black Dog is prowling.

If you have never played an instrument before but would like to try, it is never too late. For an adult beginner I suggest you start with a guitar or keyboard. Both instruments lend themselves to start-ups and can be kept in a cupboard or even taken with you. You can learn the musical notations on them and as you progress decide whether you want to proceed to the piano, do more advanced guitar work, or take up another stringed instrument. If you are attracted to another type of instrument – brass or woodwind – do not let adulthood put you off. Try them out. Once you become really interested in what you are doing it is a good idea to find yourself a teacher. You can do this through the Yellow Pages or by telephoning your local secondary school. They will put you in touch with someone who will help.

Black Dogs do not like musical instruments.

We are like a sailing ship, which has to sail through good weather and bad weather – through seas which are sometimes rough and sometimes calm. We have to keep ourselves in balance by trimming our sails to the wind, sometimes steering a more comfortable course, securing shifting cargo, and in threatening times discarding some of it.

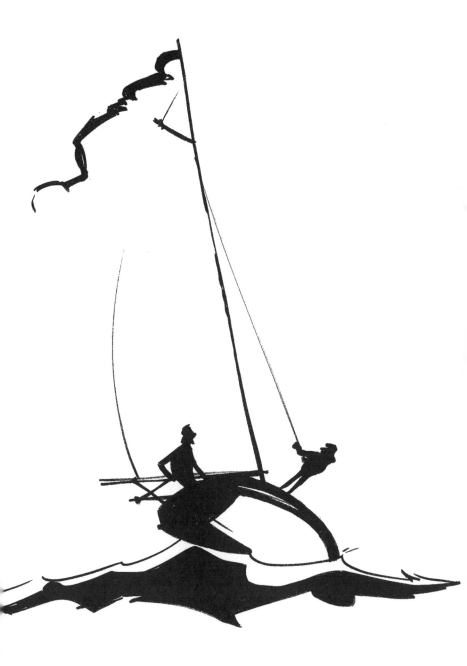

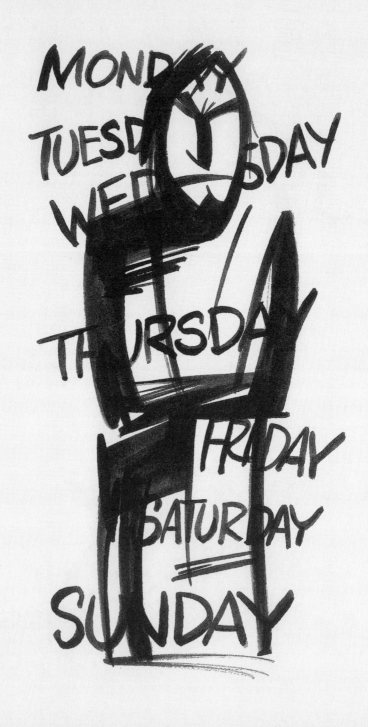

Chapter 3

Getting to Know Your Black Dog

BEFORE WE CAN CONSTRUCT A PROGRAMME for taming your Black Dog you need to sharpen your knowledge of yourself. This means becoming consciously aware of your present circumstances and lifestyle and how this is interacting with your depression. You are now going to undertake an interesting research project which will reveal to you the nature and habits of your own Black Dog.

To start with you will need to have a one-page-a-day or two-page-a-day pocket appointments diary, ideally with the hourly time slots already printed. In it I want you to record the time, circumstances and nature of your Black Dog attacks, from the moment you awaken to going to bed. There is no need to write an essay, just a few jottings are more than adequate. At the same time record what you eat and drink.

Wednesday 21/04/04

7am	*Woke up. Black Dog. Frightened of getting up. 10 mins to creep out of bed.*
	Tea, dress, toast and marmalade, coffee.
8am	*Walk 30 mins.*
9am	*Office, feeling better.*
11am	*Project meeting. Felt incompetent. Everyone else chirpy.*
1pm	*Half bottle of wine and sandwiches with the guys.*
2pm	*Weary. Long afternoon. Fearful, can't cope.*
6pm	*Two pints of beer with the guys, feeling better.*

7.30pm   Chinese takeaway, half bottle of wine.
*   Slept in front of television*
11pm   Bed. Weary and down-hearted.

Thursday 22/04/04

2am   Woke up, can't sleep. Worried about something someone
*   said yesterday about project. Credit card payment. Brain*
*   charging from one image to another. Feeling frightened.*
*   Can't stop it.*
3am   Must have dozed off.
7am   Woke up. Black Dog, frightened of getting up. Another
*   day. Hell!*

WHAT TO RECORD IN YOUR DIARY

Alcohol

There are many contributory causes of depression, irrespective
of whether the affliction is temporary or whether, like me, you
have inherited a propensity for the beast. Keep an accurate
account of *what* you drink, *how much* you drink, *when* you drink
and *why* you drink. Be honest with yourself – there is no reason
why you should not be. Nobody else will know. *(See Chapter 15)*

Food

Similarly, meal times and menus should feature in your daily
diary, as well as snacks and comfort eating. Skipping breakfast,
snacking and eating late evening meals will impair your defences
significantly. *(See Chapter 13.)* It is a good idea to have your
evening meal as early as practicable. It will reduce the
opportunity for pre-dinner drinking and give you time for a 20-
minute walk before turning in. This will help you to have a good
night's sleep.

Leisure time

Record when, how and with whom you spend your leisure time. Note down how you felt before, during and after.

Drugs

Have you started to use drugs to assuage the pain of depression? If you use drugs, keep an accurate account in your diary of what you take and when. Record what you use, how you administer it and why, e.g. feeling down, to join in with others, to relax. Also record the circumstances, e.g. in private, with friends, at a party, etc. Were you drinking alcohol at the time? Finally write down the effect, and how you feel when the effect has worn off.

> *Drug addiction is a serious problem, and outside the remit of this book. If you are relying on drugs to cope with life, then you need specialist help. See the Useful contacts section in Appendix 2.*

Your metabolic clock

Part of the brain manages our metabolism. This is called our metabolic clock. Our metabolic clocks are set at different times. For example, some people are at their most productive quite late at night, whilst others are best in the early morning. Some people, like politicians, can manage with much less sleep than others. Margaret Thatcher, it is said, managed on three or four hours' sleep each night, and Winston Churchill was the master of the cap nap and had a prodigious capacity for working long hours, despite his Black Dog.

Two friends of mine are at their most effective late at night and only need three hours' continuous sleep. In contrast, I work best in the morning, starting at 6.30 or earlier sometimes, and can find it difficult to concentrate after 2pm. I need eight hours sleep at night to be on form.

> *Record in the front of your diary those times when you are at your most productive – and use them.*

In contrast there are periods in each 24 hours when our metabolism slows down. Many people have low metabolism at between two and three in the morning, which interestingly enough is when illnesses reach their crises and when people are more likely to die. It's also when we are assailed by self-doubt and fear. You know, the dark hour before the dawn.

We experience low and slow times during the day as well.

> *Write down your low and slow times in your diary.*

Now you are starting to see how you are programmed.

Weekly and monthly digest
Each Sunday I want you to write down in your diary those features of your depression which are recurring and the current status of the things that are threatening and worrying you, like credit card payments, your partner's behaviour, salary or promotion – any of your fears. Similarly, at the end of the month write up a digest of the four weeks. You should now perceive a pattern, revealing the days, times and circumstances when the Black Dog attacks.

Each day of the week has a different character and we are more vulnerable on some days than others. 'Monday blues' is widely referred to as though the day itself was responsible, when it is usually alcoholic remorse after over-indulgence during the weekend.

I plan my Sundays with greater care than any other day. It is the one day of the week which has a certain emptiness about it – and the Black Dog likes emptiness. It is, of course, our day of rest and rehabilitation and rest is necessary for our health, but this does not mean having no purpose. We need to plan interesting but relaxing activities for it. Walking with friends or the family in the countryside. Attending church, chapel, mosque, temple or synagogue. The Sunday lunch party. Physical and competitive leisure pursuits are good occupations for Sunday but you need to plan them ahead. **Do not** make Sunday the excuse for an alcoholic binge.

It is very important to have somebody to share your interest and to keep you occupied. Just as adrenaline is the greatest antidote for depression, so inactivity and aimlessness foster the attentions of the Black Dog. Fill the subsequent hiatus with alcohol and you have a poisoned chalice, which will guarantee your demoralisation. So long drinking sessions are not a good idea.

HAS TRAUMA CONTRIBUTED TO YOUR DEPRESSION?

Trauma is a prime cause of depression. As part of this exercise in finding out about the nature of your Black Dog, read the following list of causes thoughtfully.

■ Bereavement
■ Serious disagreement with your partner, colleagues, friend, parents or children

- Separation or divorce
- Loss of trust in loved one
- Debt
- Career disappointment
- Exam stress
- Apparent failure through setting unattainable performance standards for yourself.
- Profound disappointment resulting from unrealistic life expectations.
- Redundancy and/or unemployment
- Illness (yourself or a loved one)
- Infertility
- New baby
- Accident/shock

Now underline the ones that apply to you and add any others you can think of that are not on the list.

Consider each one closely. Then ask yourself, 'Is it still with me? Is the problem still unresolved?' and write yes or no next to the ones you have underlined. That is all. This simple exercise will bring the worry, fear and uncertainty out of the cupboard of your mind. Now write the causes you've marked 'yes' in the note part of your diary. Into diary, out of mind.

WHAT TO DO NEXT

When the Black Dog is prowling again you will know the unresolved issues that are encouraging it. The sooner you can shake them out and rectify them, the sooner you will have tamed or perhaps even defeated your Black Dog. 'How on earth am I going to do that?' you may well ask.

The answer is by systematically applying the principals explained in the other sections of this manual. For the present there are two things that you can introduce immediately:

1. *Exercise. Walk for 40 minutes – now and every day. Outdoor exercise is the best immediate daily treatment for depression.*

2. *Get your adrenaline surging. Do something exciting each week and particularly at the weekend.*

Combining these two will rebalance your outlook almost immediately.

What to do with this information?

Well, being forewarned is being forearmed. When you wake up feeling weary and fearful, or are unaccountably filled with apprehension about an impending telephone call that you have to make; when you feel overwhelmed by the schedule of tasks before you; when you experience rising panic and screaming incredulity because your partner or colleague cannot immediately recognise your view point, you know that it is the Black Dog and you now know the likely causes of the Black Dog, so you are in a position to handle them and tame it.

SUMMARY

■ Purchase a one- or two-page-a-day pocket diary with times.

■ Record your productive and your low and slow times at the front.

■ Each day enter the timings and character of your Black Dog attacks.

■ Keep an account of what you drink and eat each day and the time.

■ Each weekend write up a digest of your experiences.

■ Similarly write up a digest at the end of the month.

■ From the list of underlying causes, record those which are relevant to you.

■ Look for the patterns in your experiences – they will help you understand your Black Dog, and what you need to do to tame it.

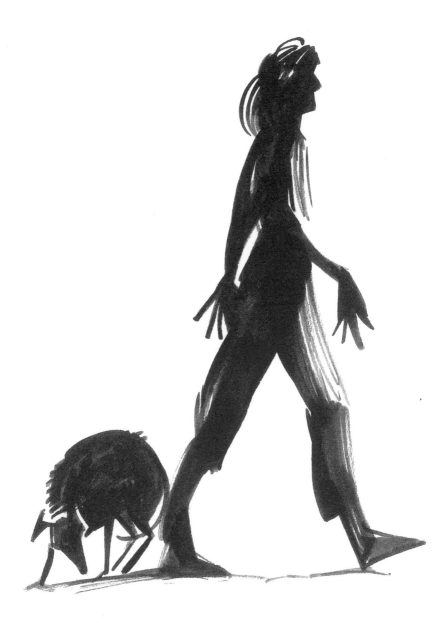

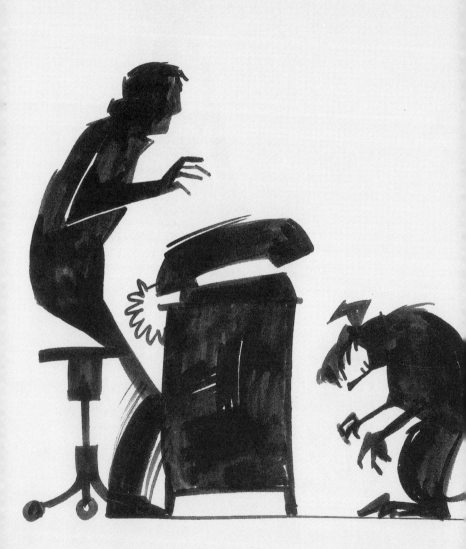

Chapter 4
Managing your life

A DEBILITATING FEATURE OF DEPRESSION IS BEING OVERWHELMED by what seems to be needed to be done each day. I say *seems* because not everything needs to be done and in any case there is only time to do so much. This lack of control magnifies apprehension and promotes panic attacks. One then finds oneself boxed into inertia by seemingly conflicting and simultaneous demands.

> *Planning each day and each week is fundamental to a happy and creative lifestyle. It is an important aspect of stress management and is an essential component in taming your Black Dog.*

We already do it occasionally, for example when we write out a shopping list or put down all the things that need to be done before going on holiday. However, we have to be more specific and selective, dare I say scientific, if we are to achieve the two prime goals of taming the Black Dog and improving our effectiveness. So where do we start? At the beginning or the end? At the end, of course. We plan our next day at the end of the present one.

PLANNING EACH DAY

There are three aspects to effective planning:

1. Make a list of everything that is waiting for you to attend to.

2. Then prioritise the urgency of the individual items, as immediate, a.m., p.m., tomorrow, any other day.

3. Now allocate time for the completion of each task, e.g.:
   a.m., three telephone calls, 5 mins each = 15 minutes
   a.m., project meeting = 30 mins
   p.m., doctor = 1 hour including travelling
   p.m., preparing supper = 30 mins
   Friday 8.30 a.m., weekly shopping, 1 hour 50 mins including journey time.

If you are a business executive you may have a secretary or PA to order your day and arrange your diary. From now on you must ensure that they enter your **personal** daily commitments before any others. Really? Yes, really.

However long your list may be, there are four items which are to be included in your diary every day without fail, and from now on are to take precedence over everything else. They are what I classify as 'standing orders' and all the other items are to be fitted round them. They are:

40 mins every morning	*walk or run and exercises (see Chapter 14)*
5 mins every morning and evening	*positive commitment habits (see Chapter 8)*

20 mins every day at midday	*meditation and auto-suggestion (see Chapters 10 and 11)*
30 mins minimum every evening	*quiet time (alone or with a friend or partner)*
once a week	*sporting activities*

I can hear all the business executives, men and women, crying that this is impractical. Everyone knows that they have to be at the beck and call of either their clients or their bosses or both, and in any event have to conform to the inflexible discipline of a big organisation. In business, their interests come last.

Think again!

Your value to your business is a function of your effectiveness. Your effectiveness in turn is a function of your capability. Your capability depends on keeping yourself physically fit and mentally alert. These five standing items do just that.

Whatever your business or occupation is, from now on you are to plan and organise it round these five standing items because **you** are the most important person in the world to those who love you and depend on you.

In a business organisation, you are a disposable item, irrespective of how elevated and powerful you may have become. **In your family you are indispensable.** Do not forget it. Charity begins and ends at home with you. The ancient meaning of charity is love.

Four reasons for planning your day the night before

1. It is easier to do it when the pressures of the day are off and
   you are relaxed. Your brain is then free to wander and you
   are able to consider what you want to accomplish as you
   write. Furthermore, in writing your thoughts down you
   effectively transfer them from your brain to paper. The result
   – worries are diminished and you are more likely to enjoy
   undisturbed sleep.

2. Visualising the actions that you are going to take and the
   results you want to achieve is best done when there is no
   residual clutter from the working day.

3. Your subconscious brain is like a highly efficient computer,
   which operates at its best while you are asleep. During that
   time it will evaluate the relative importance of the tasks that
   you have listed and prioritise them for you. Furthermore, it
   will find solutions to what the day before appeared to be
   intractable problems. It will find a way round, over or under
   the obstacles. You may also discover that it has provided you
   with original and exciting creative ideas. (See Chapter 10.)

   It is not by chance that in the past, people would often not
   make a decision until they had slept on it. They did not know
   about the subconscious. They did know, however, that if they
   asked their brain a question at night, it would more often than
   not provide them with an answer the following morning.

4. Significantly, the Black Dog cannot gain access to your
   subconscious and therefore cannot influence the evaluation of
   the solutions.

ALLOCATING TIME PERIODS

Pre-allocating a time period for the implementation of each task is not just a good forecasting procedure, it also gives the magnitude of the task a comprehensible arithmetical value. This is really helpful when the Black Dog is telling you that the task is too big for you, and you feel that you cannot cope.

When you are dreading making a telephone call

Have you come across the 20 ton telephone? That critical telephone call that you have been postponing because for some reason you are dreading making it. You balefully study the awful instrument whilst agonising about what response you are likely to receive at the other end. Will you be sufficiently on the ball to handle the other party successfully? What happens if you fail? The Black Dog is sitting in front of your desk, threatening and salivating and sweeping its tail slowly from side to side. You are irrationally afraid and the more you procrastinate the greater the threat and the weakening of your confidence.

Write down the issues and your bullet points and allocate five minutes to the call. That is all. Five minutes – that's nothing. You can handle a five-minute knockabout. **Now do it.** Take a deep breath and go. Put yourself back in control. When you put the receiver down not only will it be lighter but the space in front of your desk will have been vacated.

Putting it into perspective

You will find that the pre-allocation of time inhibits these irrational feelings and puts the size of each task into perspective. It doesn't matter whether you are suffering from an attack of the Black Dog, five minutes is still five minutes, and 30 minutes is still half an hour, although I must admit that there have been times in my life when they have seemed much longer.

Quite often there are tasks, sometimes unpleasant, sometimes simply inconvenient, from which we shy away. The more we put off dealing with them the larger they become, until they are themselves the cause of a Black Dog attack. So the lesson here is to allocate time for the completion of each task and as far as the unpleasant one is concerned – and there will be one almost every day – **DO IT NOW.**

PLANNING FOR THE UNEXPECTED

The unexpected is a feature of everyone's daily life. No matter how systematically we plan each day, week and month, something will happen to throw it out of kilter in one way or another. This feature of life has perplexed humans for time immemorial. Think of all the quotes – 'Many a slip between cup and lip'; 'Don't count your chickens before they are hatched'; 'The best laid schemes o' mice an' men gang aft a-gley'.

The point is that having a plan for the day, week and month permits you to handle contingencies. You are able to manage a new and unexpected situation. You remain in control of your life. You are in charge, irrespective of whether the changes are caused by the Black Dog or simply the unforeseeable.

After all, it may not be a disaster. It may constitute a striking opportunity or be a stroke of good fortune. Whatever, it will require a decisive response, which you can contemplate only if you are working to a plan, if you are the general commanding your affairs.

DO NOT WORK UNTIL YOU DROP

How many men and women do you know who work for hours after everyone else has left the office, only to return home numb with fatigue and apparently oblivious to the impact this is having on their partner? A director of one of the NHS's biggest areas told me that he was unable to take more than a week's holiday at any one time because if he took longer he would be unable to catch up with the accumulated paperwork. Much of his time was taken up by endless meetings, he said, and therefore he had no time for the creative, hands-on management work, for which he had a real talent. Here was a prime candidate for the Black Dog. But what can someone in such a position do about it?

As a senior manager I would have done my best to institute a procedural structure and communications network within my department which would give me the time to make best use of my talents and to think. I would have involved my staff and colleagues in the exercise and welded us all together into an integrated mutually supportive team, allowing everyone time for holidays and self-expression. If the organisational culture or the constraints of the job had prevented me from doing this I would have changed my job to preserve my sanity and protect my family life.

The Black Dog loves people whose work leaves them no time for a private life, as much as it loves those who have time on their hands. So don't do it. There are no prizes for exhaustion, but there is a penalty to pay – sometimes a devastating one!

Of course there are times when we have to be totally focussed and single minded about the work with which we are engaged. Success is not born out of idleness. Studying for an examination, preparing a live TV transmission, rehearsing for a concert, writing a business plan or managing a difficult assignment requires our total commitment and dedication. We simply cannot afford to take our eyes off the ball for a second, nor should we. Such work is creative, the short-term stress is healthy, and the reward lies in the achievement. A good antidote for Black Dog.

Whatever your circumstances, you must allocate a fixed amount of time for yourself and those who are closest to you. You need to make time for exercise, leisure activities, cultural pursuits, family life and most importantly for love. Love cannot suddenly be switched on at a whim. It is a sensitive plant and both lovers need to give it time to release itself from the detritus of a working day in order for it to blossom into affectionate intercourse. Sexual love within the security of an established relationship is a necessary and healthy ingredient for a happy life. It is a sure-fire antidote for the Black Dog's bite and it needs to be allocated time. *(See Chapter 2.)*

AVOID SETTING YOURSELF UNREALISTICALLY HIGH STANDARDS

Capable, intelligent and ambitious people have a greater propensity for depression than the general population, and it is precisely these people who often ignore or fail to appreciate the importance of working within a socially acceptable time-frame. They work intensively and set themselves unreasonably high standards of expectation and performance.

Women in commerce and the media are particularly susceptible to overdo things, perhaps because they feel the need to prove their competence to their male counterparts. They expose themselves to emotional exhaustion and sometimes isolation. This is misguided as exhaustion does not equate with success.

> *Men and women who impose on themselves very high targets for performance and try to measure up to impossibly high standards are sitting ducks for the Black Dog.*

SUMMARY

■ Not everything needs to be done in one day. List your tasks for the following day the evening before, and prioritise them.

■ Allocate a specific time for the completion of each task.

■ If you are putting off an unpleasant task, think about it in terms of how long it will take – and do it now.

■ Build into each day and week's programme periods for exercise, leisure activities, cultural pursuits, family life and love.

■ Let your subconscious work for you while you sleep.

■ Review the standards you have set yourself – are they too high?

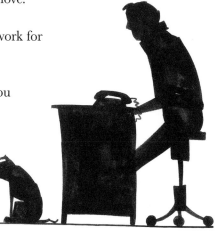

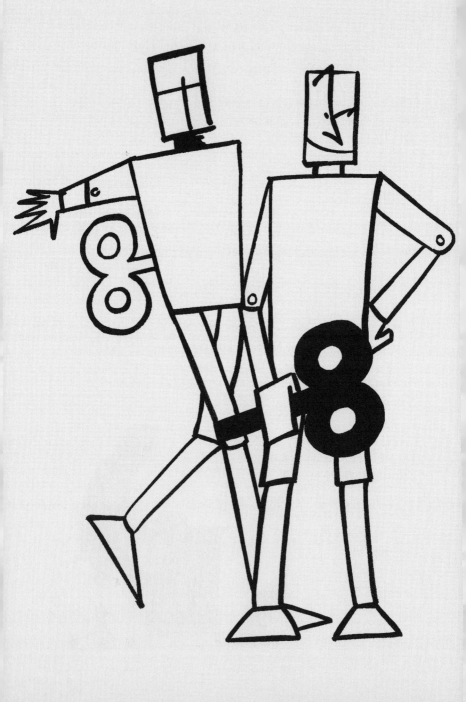

Chapter 5

Identifying and Changing Your Mental Habits

MANY OF THE THINGS WE DO EACH DAY ARE DONE OUT OF HABITS which are so well established that we do not think consciously about what we are doing. We have practised them for years and because they do not utilise intellectual capacity they permit us to do more than one thing at a time. Some of our habits are practical ones like hanging up the car keys, driving, ducking under a low beam, waking up at a particular time and attending to bodily functions. There are two other classes of habit, however, which exert powerful influences on our prospects for the success or failure of our endeavours. They are **thinking habits** – and there are good ones and bad ones. In this chapter and the next we are going to consider both and learn techniques for acquiring good positive ones to squeeze out the bad negative ones.

BAD HABITS

I am not referring to eating peas off a knife – all that will do is cut your tongue. I want to focus on the negative thinking habits which depression has cultivated in us, like low self-esteem, defeatism, fear, insularity, resentment, purposelessness, to name but a few. These negative habits are the wounds that we have suffered from the attentions of the Black Dog, over a period of time. Now we are going to heal them.

Of course, this is easier said than done – it always is, isn't it? The problem is that over a period of time we have become actually comfortable in our introverted self-pitying state of mind and use it as a defence mechanism. When we wake up with a bad attack of Black Dog, and curl into a foetal ball whimpering to ourselves that we want to die or cannot face the day, we are actually enjoying ourselves. During the day a disappointment, or seemingly another failure, drives us back into this self-indulgent hole and probably makes us think about a slug of alcohol to numb the pain.

In overcoming these negative thinking habits, we also have to contend with an over-powering weariness, itself a symptom of depression, which saps our vitality and undermines our ability to cope. Drinking to obtain short-term relief is very seductive, but magnifies the weariness and can make us suicidal. *(See Chapter 15.)*

There doesn't seem to be much going for us, does there? Well, as General Slim said at a low point in the Burma campaign, 'Things are never quite as bad or quite as good as you think they are.' Smile, then – things could be worse. The fact that you have arrived at this point of the book indicates a determination on your part to tame your Black Dog. You will be cheered up no end as you practise the positive habits and squeeze out the negative ones.

HOW HEALTHY ARE YOUR ATTITUDES?

The following is a list of seven negative attitudes. Underline those that you feel may apply to you at the moment. If you have other more exotic ones, put them down – and let me know what they are, I might want to keep one myself.

- Expectation of failure   'Everything always goes wrong for me.'
- Self-criticism   'I'm stupid or lazy or both.'
- Low self-esteem   'I've achieved nothing compared to other people. I'm worthless.'
- Guilt   'It's all my fault.'
- Fear   'What if… ?'
- Emptiness   'I really don't care what happens.'
- Lack of purpose   'It's all pointless. Why bother?'

Underline those that are dominating your attitude at the moment. Think round them for a bit and ask yourself why. Leave it at that. We are going to come back to them later.

Each of our emotional habits operate with varying intensity according to our circumstances, but usually only one powerful emotion dominates at a time. When you espy a fellow chatting up a pretty girl over a bottle of claret in a corner of a bistro there is little doubt which one is dominating his and you may assume that it is wholly positive.

In contrast, negative attitudes also pop up and dominate us. This is not all bad news, because it permits us to focus the whole of our intellect on knocking one out at a time with a shot of positive thinking. How? Read on, the best is yet to come. No, don't make a grab for the claret decanter yet. You will find, devised especially for you, positively charged ammunition with which to neutralise the negative characteristics cultivated by your Black Dog.

FOUNDATION DAILY HABITS – KNOCKING OUT NEGATIVE ATTITUDES WITH POSITIVE THOUGHTS

To start with there are two habits which I want you to practise. Make them an automatic start and finish to every day and a permanent part of your make-up. Afterward I am going to help you to create your own positive thinking habits designed to knock out your particular negative and defeatist thoughts.

Habit number 1 – plan and prioritise

Each evening list in your diary all the tasks that need to be done and prioritise them according to their urgency. (See Chapter 4.)

Habit number 2 – four principles every day

Read, learn and consider in depth the following four fundamental principles in terms of your own life today. Write them down in your diary and commit them to your memory.

Recite them to yourself every morning, noon and evening, on the way to work and on your way home and whenever the Black Dog strikes.

First principle: Everything in our world is changing – continually

These words are making changes to you now as you read. The world – your world, my world – is different today than it was yesterday. New things are happening, opinions are changing, people are entering and leaving our lives, we are constantly saying hello or goodbye to something or somebody. New opportunities and threats enter our lives every day.

Second principle: Your past is dead

Nothing in it can be changed. There will certainly be things that you have learnt from it, that is why we study history. But your past is wholly unresponsive to contemplation, so do not waste your time ruminating. All that does is to provide nourishment for the Black Dog. Look forwards.

Third principle: Your time is finite.
Do not waste it. Every minute you dwell in the past you are denying yourself time in the present. Make the most of the here and now.

Fourth principle: What you do today creates your future.
Your thoughts and actions create your life tomorrow, next week, next month. What you do today will affect other people's futures as well. Your actions in the present have the potential to bring happiness, joy, success and freedom to yourself and to others.

Write the statement below in your diary or on a piece of card to use as a bookmark with your name in the space.

I .... understand that all things change and that I can change all things in my life. My actions today will decide my future.

Got it? Good, hang on to it. Now we can proceed by creating some good positive thinking habits specially for you.

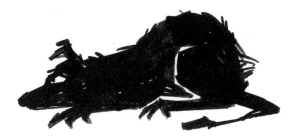

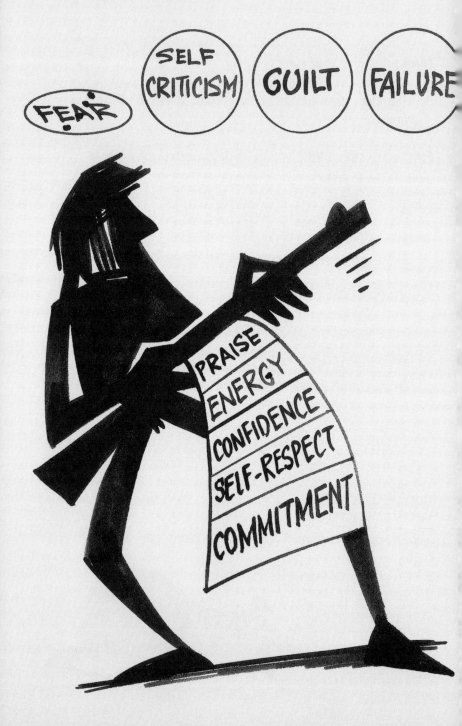

sleeping bags
loo
gaz + tube
+ clip
bowls.

check
tent
airbed

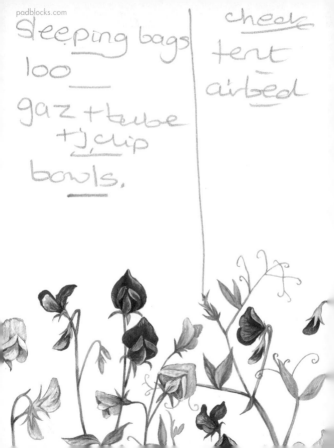

Chapter 6

Creating Your Own Personal Commitment Habits – Finding Out About Yourself

FIRSTLY I WANT YOU TO ISOLATE THE NEGATIVE ATTITUDES that your Black Dog has cultivated for you and also the characteristics you like least in yourself. These are your principal targets which we are going to knock out with fresh, positive attitudes.

YOUR DOMINANT NEGATIVE ATTITUDES

Below is the list of negative attitudes that you examined in Chapter 5, plus a few more. Add any extra ones that you found. Read them through and underline the three dominant ones, the ones that you feel apply to you most. These are the first negative, corrosive attitudes that you are about to deal with. It's called target acquisition and you are going to get good at it. If you have more than three dominant ones, don't worry, you can deal with the others in due course. For the present I only want you to knock out three negatives at a time. With practice and experience you will be able to handle more.

Your negative targets

- Expectation of failure
- Self-criticism
- Low self-esteem
- Guilt
- Fear

- Emptiness
- Lack of purpose
- Feeling useless
- Feeling unloved
- Irritability
- Selfishness
- Weariness
- Being defeatist
- Can't be bothered

Add your own little treasures here!

Think about each of the three that you have selected and consider whether you know the causes behind them. For example, if you are lazy, is it because you lack vitality, or have no one to motivate you, or that you have no purpose in life, or is it a combination of all three? If you feel unloved, is it because you are ashamed of yourself for some reason, that you have isolated yourself from family and friends, or that you are resentful and bitter over something in your past life?

Try to consider each attitude honestly, but without adding further to your self-criticism habit.

The point is that half of your battle is won if you can put your finger on the underlying causes. Don't worry if, for the moment, you cannot find a reason – you will, and in the meantime, with the help of positive thoughts, you can start to diminish them, and tame your Black Dog.

Now continue and enjoy some sunshine.

I have made up a list of positive attributes, for you. Take some time in considering them and again add any of your own.

Positive attributes

- Anticipation of success
- Praise
- Self-respect
- Clear conscience
- Confidence
- Fulfilment
- Purposefulness
- Feeling worthy
- Feeling loved
- Patience
- Thoughtfulness
- Energy
- Winning
- Commitment

Now move on to see why these particular positive attributes are so special.

They are the positive antonyms – the opposites – of the negative attitudes in the previous list. And they constitute the ammunition for your knock-out gun.

Targets	*Ammunition*
Expectation of failure	Anticipation of success
Self-criticism	Praise
Low self-esteem	Self-respect
Guilt	Clear conscience
Fear	Confidence
Emptiness	Fulfilment
Lack of purpose	Purposefulness
Feeling useless	Feeling worthy
Feeling unloved	Feeling loved
Irritability	Patience
Selfishness	Thoughtfulness
Weariness	Energy
Being defeatist	Winning
Can't be bothered	Commitment
Miserable	Cheerful
Depressed	Happy

For the three dominant negatives that you have underlined, now underline the opposite – the positive – for each one.

If you have added any negatives of your own, see if you can think of their opposites, and add them to the list of positives.

A question for you: Why do you think the last two characteristics in each column are separated from the rest? No, nothing is missing and it's not a printing error. No, it's not because they are more important than the rest. It is because they are the sum total of the other 14.

The result of holding onto your negative attitudes is misery and depression.
The result of adopting positive attitudes is cheerfulness and happiness.

Now move on to the next chapter to find out how to go about making these positive attitudes a reality for you.

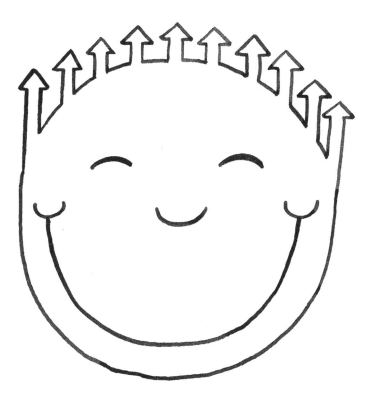

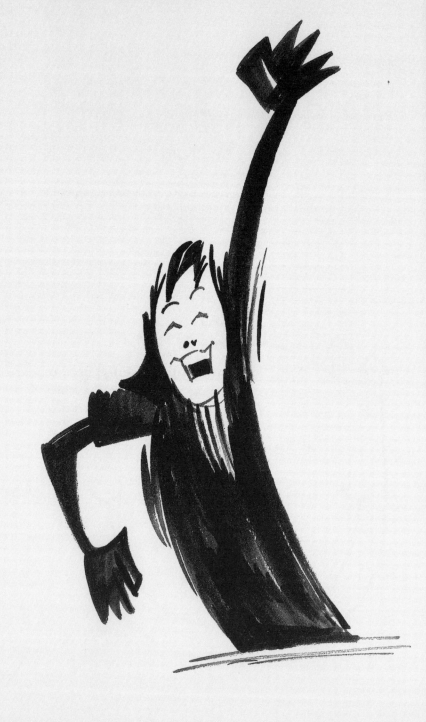

Chapter 7

Creating Your Own Personal Commitment Habits – Taking Action

SELF-CRITICISM

When properly used, self-criticism is part of a self-learning mechanism. Reversing your car into a wall is not an accident, it is the result of inattention and a quick self-scold at the time is appropriate. Arriving late for an appointment because you did not allocate sufficient time for the journey justifies a self-scolding.

However, **irrational and unjustified self-criticism inflicts more and more damage to our self-respect each time we do it** – and it is cumulative. You know the sort of thing: 'Trust me to get in the slow lane – story of my life.' 'I could have gone for the later train – only someone as daft as me would be up at this time in the morning.' 'Mary wasn't very responsive last night. Must be something I said.' 'What a fool for trying to do the DIY myself, should have got an expert in, now I've made a right mess of it – typical!' And so on…

These examples may provoke a self-admonishing smile, but when they represent a permanent attitude of mind towards yourself they will undermine your morale. Like anything rotten they need to be eradicated, along with the bad, bad habit of making fun of yourself, in order to pre-empt criticism or to raise a cheap laugh.

LOW SELF-ESTEEM FOLLOWS SELF-CRITICISM

Remember some of those old wise and tested adages? 'If you can't say something good about someone, don't say anything.' 'Always look for the best in others.' If these sayings are appropriate for how you should think and talk about everyone else then they are appropriate for **you**. So if you have nothing good to say about yourself, shut up. From this moment on, whenever you have a self-critical thought, kill it with the words **'Shut up!'** Then summon up a success thought about yourself and say **'Now that's good.'** Keep a bank of good thoughts ready to be used on these occasions:

- Recall the help you have given to other people.
- Admire your attainments.
- Warm to your love for someone and their love for you.
- Relish your successes.
- Think about your current objective.
- Focus on your purpose.
- Remember the people you admire.
- Say aloud, 'I am succeeding and I am proud of me.'
- Look forwards, not backwards.

Whenever you complete a task successfully or achieve a goal, stop, take time out and congratulate yourself – because you deserve it!

CREATING DAILY POSITIVE COMMITMENT HABITS

Every commitment is written in the present tense as though it is a current reality. Using the imperative of 'I will' does not work. Remember the third principle from Chapter 4? It says what you do in the present decides you future – and that goes for the ideas that you express.

We are now going to create daily positive commitment habits to deal with four of the most common negative attitudes that are food and drink to the Black Dog.

Self-criticism
Let's devise a daily positive commitment to kill this joker.

What is the positive antonym of self-criticism? Refer to page 46 to find out. Yes, it is **praise**. So compose your daily habit statement round it:

> *I .... have tamed the Black Dog. I recognise my achievements, visualise them and I congratulate myself. I feel good about myself and others. I remember that if I cannot say something positive about someone I say nothing, and that goes for me as well.* **The rule is: Praise or silence.**

Write it in your diary and recite it six times each morning and six times each evening and whenever you find you are about to put yourself down or make fun of yourself. **Praise or shut up!**

Low self-esteem

Follow the same procedure. Refer to page 46 and you will find that the antonym is **self-respect**.

> *I* .... *am justifiably proud of myself.*
> *I recall my achievements and successes today, which are*
> .... *and I am pleased with my*
> *endeavour. I see the best in everyone, including myself. I am*
> *confident in my ability to manage my affairs successfully and to*
> *help others.* **I love myself just as I love**
> .... [name of loved one(s)]. **Yes I do.**

Defeatism and expectation of failure

Whenever we have an expectation of failure we are dead in the water and like all wrecks we are a constant danger to others as well as ourselves. It is a negative attitude of mind, which is infectious if it is not eradicated. In the armed services the utterance of defeatist thoughts is an offence. It is described as 'spreading alarm and despondency'. During the Second World War, defeatism was recognised as being so dangerous to national morale that to be heard expressing it was an imprisonable offence and a court martial offence in the services. Today it appears in different guises, such as being 'risk-averse', and scuttles many good ideas and potentially successful projects, both personal and professional. So it would seem sensible to rid ourselves of it PDQ.

First you must decide what is the cause of your defeatism. Is it because you are trying to do something for which you have neither the skill nor the talent? Have you for the moment just had one setback too many? Is it because your life seems to be in such a mess that you are overwhelmed by the complexity of your misfortune? Are you afflicted by depression more profoundly than usual or is it a combination of all these possible causes? Or is it that you are being 'wet', self-indulgent and feeling sorry for yourself? If it's the latter don't bother reading further – just get up, get out and go for a six-mile walk.

Refer to the causes of your depression in your diary notes and see which ones are promoting defeatism.

Now consider whether these causes are being imposed on you by an external force or whether they are an attitude of mind.

If you are drinking or taking drugs you have the power to rectify it. You may need help but it is in your power to make a change. *(See Chapter 15.)*

If you have had one bashing too many and your life is in ruins, following the procedures in this book will help you to get on your feet again. But for now refer again to the four principles on page 40 and read them out aloud six times. Go on, do it now. Got it? Now look at your present predicament through the lens of these four principles and consider carefully how it now appears. Read them out again while you think over your misfortune and notice how hope starts to make a timid appearance. Slowly but surely its flame will strengthen. It will grow into faith and finally confidence. So let's get going. Let's defeat defeatism.

The past cannot be undone but there are steps that you can take to salvage what is valuable. The biggest change that you can make is to plot a new course and embark on it.

So now let's design a personal commitment habit.

> *I* .... *am **winning**. Defeatism is an attitude of mind, which I have extinguished with purpose. I anticipate success in all my endeavours. **I am winning.***

Fear

Fear is a necessary response to danger, it prompts us to fight or run away from a physical threat. But when fear becomes an all-pervasive part of our everyday lives, it can paralyse us. We can develop a habit of living in a constant state of irrational fear.

How can we start to deal with this fear, and put it back into perspective? Yes, we design a personal commitment habit.

> *I* ....*understand that irrational fear is an attitude of mind. I am in control of my life. When I am frightened I write down the causes and deal with them immediately. **I do it NOW. I fear naught.** I am the general commanding my life.*

Your own particular personal commitment habits

Once you have established these four daily commitment habits, and they have had time to take effect, you can move on and add some more of your own, using the first four as examples of how to construct them.

Take each of the three positive attitudes that you underlined in the previous chapter – the opposites of the negatives that you underlined. You are now going to construct a daily commitment round each one.

If the ones you underlined were the ones we have already written statements for above – great, keep going with these. Alternatively, write your own more personal versions of them, using words that are particularly powerful and effective for you.

Whichever negative attitudes you have chosen to deal with next, make the statements **succinct** and **positive**. Write them in the **present tense** as though they have already happened.

INCREASING THE EFFECTIVENESS OF YOUR DAILY POSITIVE COMMITMENT HABITS

You now have two foundation habits (see Chapter 6) and at least four positive commitment habits, which you must read aloud six times every morning and six times last thing at night – irrespective of how tired you may be. The effectiveness of this exercise depends on three things: repetition, continuity and commitment.

> *Say the positive commitment statements aloud with conviction – even shout them, if possible. It enhances their effectiveness if you hear yourself saying what you are committing to.*

However, you do not have to stop doing everything else whilst you are practising them. A particularly good time to recall them is on your walk. Call them up when you are travelling on the train (it probably wouldn't be a good idea to shout them in these circumstances!) or driving – keep a copy of them in the glove compartment in your car.

How long will it take for them to be effective?

The fact that you are doing something positive has an immediately elevating effect. Novelty adds to the interest, and the other procedures in this book will accelerate the effectiveness of your daily positive commitment habits. It will take about three months for them to become established in your psyche. However, you can accelerate the procedure and increase the depth of mental influence by combining them with your meditation and auto-suggestion. *(See Chapter 9.)*

This is where your daily diary comes in again. Write down on each page the commitment habits that you are going to practise each day for the coming month and tick them off each evening when you are writing your task list for the next day. (See Chapter 4.)

SUMMARY

- Make copies of the four main positive commitment habits and keep them in a place where you will see them every day.

- Recite them six times every morning when you wake up and every evening before you go to sleep, no matter how tired you are.

- Recite them when you are walking, driving or travelling on the train or bus.

- Keep a programme in your diary.

■ Once these four are established, refer to the negative and undesirable traits that you have underlined on page 43 and select the dominant three.

■ Turn to page 46 and write down the positive antonyms (opposite traits).

■ Following the examples, construct a commitment statement in the present tense for each one.

■ Make it simple and succinct.

■ Include these in your daily routine.

■ Success depends on repetition, continuity and commitment.

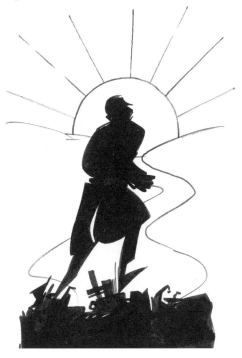

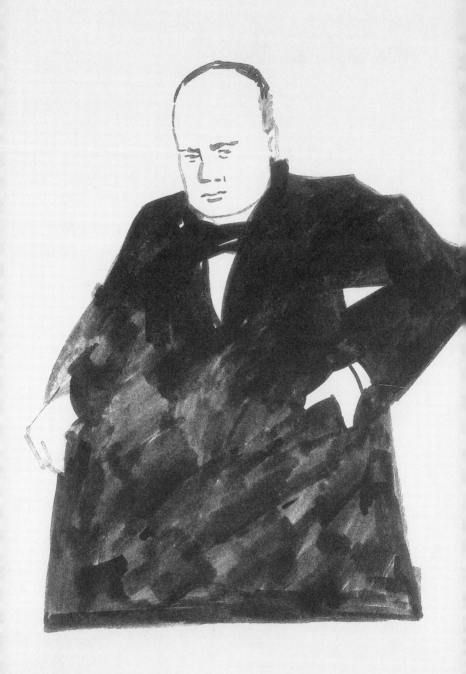

Chapter 8
Using a Role Model

I ADOPTED DIFFERENT ROLE MODELS AT DIFFERENT TIMES IN MY LIFE. Each one fulfilled my specific needs at a particular juncture in my life. They included my parents for their love and commitment to being of service to other people. My regiment's one time commanding officer, for his determination, leadership, courage and care. My editorial director for showing me the beauty of the English language, his vocabulary, intellect and charm. My governor during my merchant banking days, for his patience, understanding, confidence, wit and dignity. Finally, my dear American mentor in television, for his intelligence, quiet perception, ability to make complicated issues simple and his unfailing courtesy.

WINSTON CHURCHILL, MY ROLE MODEL

I chose Winston Churchill as my role model for taming the Black Dog because he did just that. He had an unquenchable spirit to rise above disappointments, misjudgement and failures – at times amounting almost to public disgrace. He was our greatest prime minister but might not have been if he had succumbed to the Black Dog during the time he was cast out into the political wilderness in the 1930s.

His example seemed to me to offer everyone – but particularly people living with depression – justifiable expectation for the fruitful outcome of our lives. He said that he was aware of walking with destiny throughout his life. So do we in our lives. Never forget it.

It was he who called his depression the Black Dog and is the inspiration behind this book.

I would like you to read the following excerpt from one of his early speeches, which I have used to start this book. He delivered it in a speech to his constituents in Dundee in 1915, only five days after having been sacked as first Lord of the Admiralty by Asquith, his own prime minister and friend, with all the incredulous pain it must have inflicted on him. He might well be addressing you and me today.

Then turn again to your task. Look forward, do not look backward. Gather afresh in heart and spirit all the energies of your being, bend anew together for a supreme effort. The times are harsh, the need is dire, the agony seems infinite but the power of commitment and perseverance hurled united into the conflict will be irresistible.

Because it was a war speech I have altered a couple of words in the last sentence without changing the meaning or focus. The unaltered passage appears in Appendix 1.

In moments of deep depression it has resonated through my mind. I hope this small historical divergence will motivate you, as well, to look forward not backwards and help you to find an appropriate role model to help you tame your Black Dog.

CHOOSING YOUR OWN ROLE MODEL

Following these examples I want you to do the same. A word of warning here: you must know why you respect the person you choose and why he or she is appropriate. If you admire David Beckham for his outstanding sportsmanship, leadership and sense of fair play, his devotion to his family and work for charity, then he might be a good candidate for your role model, but don't just choose him because he's a good-looking rich celebrity you've read about in the papers. I chose Winston Churchill specifically to help me with depression because I came to know him well through his writings and the biographies that have been published about him. Most importantly I shared his affliction – the Black Dog.

Consider all the people you know quite a lot about and choose the one you would most like to be. He or she can be a friend, acquaintance, philanthropist, military or political leader, community worker, artist, etc. Write down in the note part of your diary the positive features you admire in him or her.

> *A note here. If you do not have an acquaintance whom you really admire then it's time to take a critical look at the company you are keeping. A very old adage says 'Show me your friends and I'll tell you what you are.'*

Now consider whom you should adopt as your own role model – choose the person who is most appropriate to your present circumstances. When the Black Dog is barking, summon him or her up and visualise how he or she would deal with your current situation. What would their advice to you be? What words of encouragement might they give you? What action would they take?

SUMMARY

- Role models can help us in difficult times.

- Choose a role model, someone you admire and respect.

- When you're under attack from the Black Dog, visualise how this person would deal with your situation.

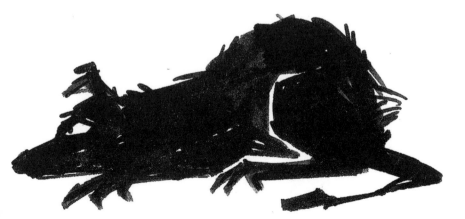

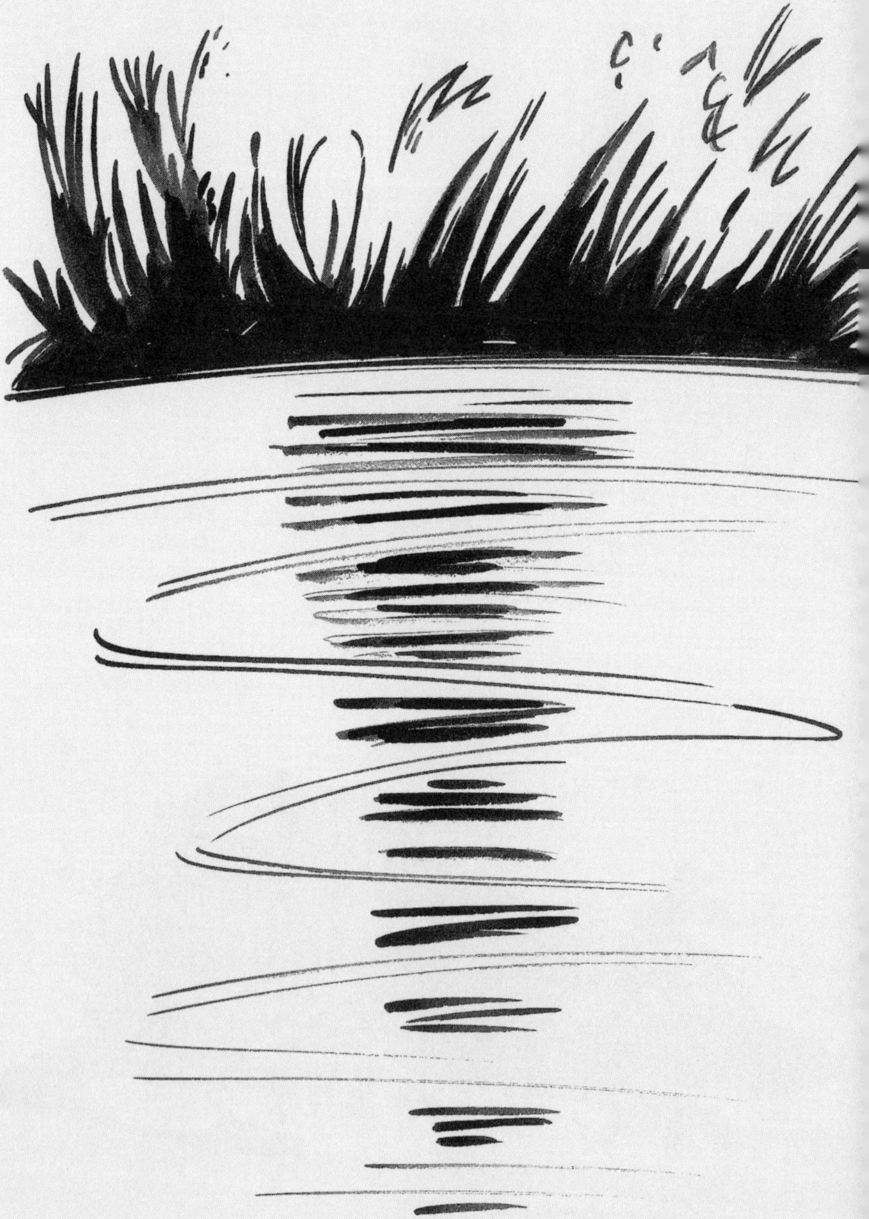

Chapter 9
Using Your Subconscious Mind

THERE ARE THREE WAYS OF USING YOUR SUBCONSCIOUS to enhance your mental effectiveness and to combat the effects of depression.

■ The first is **meditation**, which physically relaxes you while refreshing your brain and allowing it freedom to come up with inspirational ideas.

■ The second is **auto-suggestion**, whereby you use the subconscious to help you establish positive thinking habits. *(See Chapters 6 and 7, and page 71 of this chapter.)*

■ The third is in **problem solving**, whereby you write down whatever you need to deal with the following day and allow the subconscious to come up with solutions while you sleep. *(See Chapter 4.)*

USING MEDITATION

I am starting with meditation because you will find the other two applications easier to understand and carry out once you can meditate. If you have never tried to do this you are in for a treat because, although it needs daily practice, you will feel an improvement in your sense of well-being quite quickly. Furthermore, you can do it anywhere, literally anywhere.

Whenever I am driving on the motorway and start to feel tired I pull off at a service station or a junction where I find a lay-by or country lane and do 15 or 20 minutes meditation. That's all – no more than 20 minutes is sufficient to completely refresh me. You can learn to switch off for up to 20 minutes on a train, aircraft or in your office. It's a real benefit before a late afternoon meeting and it can transform your attitude of mind when you sense the incipient weariness of an approaching Black Dog attack. Of course, if you have a quiet room into which you can withdraw that is a bonus.

Meditation does not involve you emulating the role of a Himalayan guru, although this is where it started, nor does it involve you losing consciousness or falling asleep. You are always in absolute control of your faculties and capable of responding immediately to a threat or emergency. You remain totally aware of what is happening around you but you are able to detach yourself from it.

Trying it out
A CD version of this procedure is obtainable – see appendix 2. Patrick Ellverton.

So let's proceed. To start with I am going to ask you to find a quiet room somewhere where you can be alone. Sit down on a chair and check that your posture is erect but relaxed, your back is supported and that your head is squarely on your shoulders. It's a good idea to support it with cushions but not absolutely necessary if you are sitting erect. It does not need to be an armchair. Indeed, when I was first introduced to meditation we sat on upright dining chairs.

During your session of meditation you will remain fully aware of what is taking place around you – a car drawing up outside the window, someone talking in an adjoining room or a door opening and closing – but because you have detached yourself from their world for the time being you can choose to be unaffected by it.

Just one exception – the telephone. Most of us have an instant recall mechanism to the ringing of a telephone. Ensure that you are away from the sound of a telephone – unplug the telephone if it's nearby, and for goodness sake switch off your mobile. Suddenly being called back may not be harmful but I tell you it's one hell of a shock and undoes the good work already done.

Now take on board the fact that the next 20 minutes in your life are sacrosanct. They are dedicated to you alone. You are completely detached from the world around you. Note the word 'detached' not isolated. It is your decision as to when you rejoin the madding crowd. In meditation you remain in control.

Meditation is a simple, pure and natural process by which you allow yourself to drift downwards into a state of stillness, tranquillity and peace. It must not be forced and is thus different from relaxation techniques where we consciously impose a relaxed state of body and mind on ourselves. However, I have found that when I have been suffering from an attack of Black Dog it is helpful to start with the deep breathing technique we use in relaxation.

As we drift down to pure consciousness we enter a state of suspended animation and our conscious and subconscious minds become very close. Once in this state we do nothing. We just float until it is time to return. It is in this state of perfect stillness and balance that our stressed out minds and bodies are repaired and refreshed.

■ Now that you are sitting comfortably and erect, you can relax yourself physically. First wiggle your toes, then put tension into your calf muscles and relax them. Now tense your thigh muscles once or twice and relax them. Pull in your belly muscles and relax them. Now move to your finger and arm muscles, tensing each of them two or three times and relaxing them. Do the same with your shoulder muscles and finally and most importantly your neck muscles. Twist your head gently from side to side. Lift your chin and allow it to drop onto your chest, then swivel it round until all the tension has drained away from the back of your neck.

And a word here to you clever guys who are saying to yourselves 'I've done all this before. I know all about relaxing and I didn't buy this book to read what I already know.' Well, shut up. The value is not in the individual techniques, all of which have been utilised for generations, but in the cumulative effect of the whole programme.

■ Now start to inhale very slowly and deeply. Imagine the fresh clean air going down to your arms to your fingers. Down your legs to your toes and refreshing the whole of your chest cavity with life-stimulating air. As you near the peak of your intake visualise how, as you exhale, any tension in your body is blown away with the air.

■ Now breath in a bit more until your chest is bursting with air. A bit more, more, more… hold it. Now let go. Forcefully exhale until your lungs are completely empty, and as you do see the stress from your muscles expelled like coils of burnt fried onions or metal swarf from a lathe and blown away to the far corner of the room.

■ Now relax and breath quietly for a minute or so, because this technique uses up energy and you need to rest between each try. Repeat this twice more – three times in all – to become physically relaxed and ready to clear out your brain in the same way.

■ The next time as you slowly inhale imagine the clean air collecting together every weary thought and worry in your mind. Hold it, hold it. Now forcefully exhale, blowing every negative thought, every atom of weariness into the far corner of the room and leaving your brain empty and content. Do this once more and you can begin your meditation.

■ Now just be still and become aware of it. Visualise emptiness. Some people at this stage, after a few sessions, see a sort of white light. Concentrate on it. Now think about closing down your brain and becoming still and full of peace. Tranquillity starts to embrace your mind and body.

■ Now allow yourself to drift down, down, down as though you were in the most beautiful warm sea. Look up and see the underneath of the surface waves which are the stresses and threats of your working life and the fears of your depression. Leave them behind. Release yourself from your restricting conscious life. Drift away from them. Feel free. Free from your physical self. Free from every thought and idea and influence.

■ You will begin to experience total tranquillity and be completely at peace with yourself. Your breathing become shallow and your pulse will slow down and so will your blood pressure. Your metabolism will have slowed down to such an extent that your body and mind will be benefiting from a more reinvigorating rest than if you were asleep.

■ You can stay here in this state as long as you choose, but if you looked at your watch before embarking on the practice and gave yourself 20 minutes for the whole session you will begin to feel a desire to get going again after 15 minutes. Don't resist it but do not rush the process of returning. Let yourself slowly and lazily drift towards the surface of your conscious existence, taking in one or two sighs or deeper breaths on the way up. That's all it is.

What about going to sleep?

A word of warning here: avoid going to sleep if you can. Often one feels so relaxed and contented during meditation that one wants to drop off. Resist it if you can because if you go to sleep you may feel groggy when you wake up, while if you remain awake in meditation you will feel great when you finish meditating. You derive the greatest benefit from meditation when you are awake.

If you are really sleepy, after lunch for example, find an armchair, support yourself with cushions and sleep for 20 or 30 minutes. Busy people with long working days, like politicians, have always improved their productivity by having a siesta after lunch, but it is not meditation.

When to meditate

When and how often should you meditate? Pure meditation should be practised once a day, every day. Practice makes perfect and the benefits you derive increase as you become more adept.

The best times are before you become tired and when you are wide awake. For example, after dressing each morning at home, on the train, before lunch or in the evenings about 5 p.m. You can also use meditation to refresh yourself before a taxing meeting, or during a break from driving if you're getting dangerously tired.

AUTO-SUGGESTION – THE POWER OF WORDS

You can accelerate the effect of daily commitment habits *(see Chapters 6 and 7)*, particularly the ones that you have created yourself, by incorporating them in the process of becoming meditative. On no account should you consider this to be a replacement for the conscious job of reciting your daily commitment habits six times each morning and evening. The meditative process addresses your subconscious and in so doing, super-charges the effectiveness of the repetitive conscious habit.

Using words to give a positive message to your subconscious

Let us take as an example two negative traits that you are trying to replace with positive ones in your daily commitments. Let us take **weariness** and **being defeatist**. What are their positive antonyms? Well, don't wait for me to tell you, get back to page 46 and find out yourself.

Back again and got it? Good. Well if your reference work is as good as mine, the answer should be **energy** or **energetic** and **winning**. Think about them deeply. Do some imagineering and see yourself at this moment full of energy and succeeding in cheerfully driving through the obstacles that are currently insurmountable in your life. Now hold on to this dynamic image of yourself but let it settle quietly, and join together the two words into one so that they begin to constitute a complete idea, a whole image of yourself in your mind. You can play around with the words, or come up with others that you prefer, to convey the same idea.

It is not mandatory to make up composite words. It just makes it easier, I have found, when you begin to handle more than one concept at a time. After a week of establishing the first concept you can introduce a second while still operating the first. A week later you can introduce a third composite.

Now create a composite word that describes the image in your mind. How about **winnergetic**? Or **getwin** (with a soft g)? Choose one of these or make up your own, but adopt the one that best represents what you want to be. This is now your power word – let it settle and see yourself responding to the composite meaning of the word.

I'm full of energy and I'm winning.

Yes, you are!

Meditating on your power-word
Now begin your meditation procedure. Tense each of your muscle groups and relax them, starting with your toes and finishing with your neck muscles. Now the breathing. Deep breath in, in, in, in, hold it… Now let go, expelling every bit of tension in your body including that bit you didn't think you had. See it pile up in the far corner of the room like twisted burnt onions or metal swarf from a lathe. Finally the last deep breath and fill your head with fresh cleansing oxygen and then blow out and with it every thought in your mind.

Now let your mind and body rest in relaxation and quietly call back **winnergetic**. Let it arrive in its own time and also let the picture of its effect on you come into focus, like a photograph in a development tank. Slowly but surely it appears with ever greater clarity.

Now start to count yourself down to the lowest levels of consciousness by slowly and quietly in your mind counting from one to 20, and visualising yourself sinking, deeper and deeper and deeper towards tranquillity, and suspended animation. Take your **winnnergetic** image of yourself with you. Hold it, embrace it, as you descend the ladder of consciousness until you reach security and peace at number 20. Just stay there with **winnergetic**.

After a time, usually about 15 minutes or a bit less, you will begin to feel restless. Your buoyancy is returning, so start to slowly float towards the surface of your full consciousness. Hold on to **winnergetic** and at 15 repeat:

I have the energy to win.

Again at 12, and at 10. At six open your eyes, take a deep breath and feel good. Now repeat **winnergetic**, **energy to win** with each of the remaining numbers to one. The eyes wide open, a deep breath of satisfaction and a big smile. And what then? Forgotten already?

Yes, a big pat on the back. Self-congratulations to be given generously.

I won! I did it! Yes, I am winning and I am ready to go. I am proud of myself.

ACCELERATING THE EFFECTIVENESS OF YOUR POSITIVE COMMITMENT HABITS

You can apply this procedure to two daily positive habits at a time. For example, look back to Chapter 6, page 46, for the positive antonyms of self-criticism and low self-esteem – **praise** and **self-respect**. Make up a composite word, the meaning of which you can visualise. How about **praispect** or **respraise**? Or you could play around with the words and make up your own.

Choose the one with which you are most comfortable and while murmuring it, summon up a picture of yourself – quietly proud and confident in your achievements with the programme in this book, and full of love and admiration for yourself and your loved ones. Got it? Let the image mature in your mind and secure it. Now, while holding it and murmuring your key word, embark on your trip to tranquillity.

Count yourself down and at 20 rest there, nurturing the vision until you become restless. Don't resist, gently count yourself back again, repeating your key word aloud at 15 and then at 12 and at eight a deep breath and at six open your eyes and enjoy the rest of the return journey, while experiencing a growing feeling of warmth and confidence.

I am full of self-respect and give myself the praise that I richly deserve.

By following this example you can now compose your own composite words for the personal positive commitment habits that you have created for yourself – and use them to help you tame the Black Dog.

SUMMARY

- You can access your subconscious mind through meditation and auto-suggestion.

- Use the meditation technique described here to calm, refresh and uplift yourself.

- Use the power of words to help develop the positive traits you have chosen for yourself.

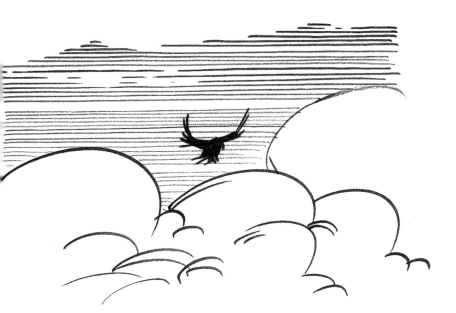

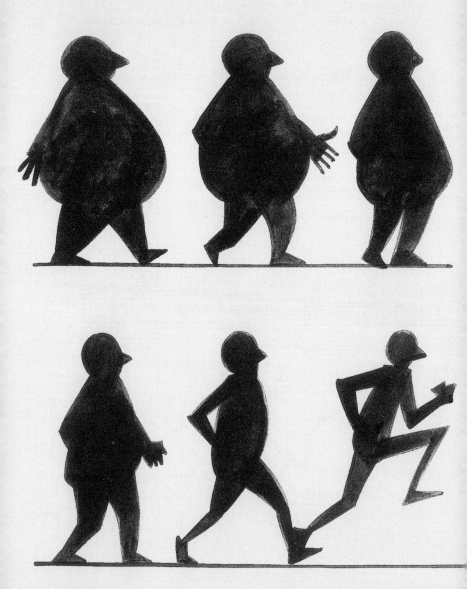

Chapter 10
Boosting Your Vitality

THE PURPOSE OF THIS SECTION IS TO HELP YOU TO WITHSTAND
Black Dog attacks.

> *The most powerful weapon in our natural armoury for taming the*
> *Black Dog is vitality.*

Vitality has three constituents – **nourishment, exercise and
rest.** The balanced combination of these three will ensure that
a reserve of energy is available to defeat depression and for most
people to recover altogether. I say 'most' because you will
remember that some of us have inherited a propensity for
depression and will need to use all the strategies described in this
book to help us throughout our lives.

YOUR POWER-TO-WEIGHT RATIO

Energy depends on getting one's power-to-weight ratio right.
People who are overweight consume energy intended for real
living, simply in moving their imperial carcasses from one place
to another. There is nothing left for real endeavour and
enjoyment.

This is a critical element in the vicious downward spiral of
demoralisation. It goes like this. People who do not eat the right
food have insufficient energy to exercise. People who do not
exercise put on weight. People who do not eat the right food and

do not take exercise become obese. Contrary to popular belief, overweight people are not generally happy bunnies and they have a much greater propensity for depression than others.

Similarly, people who deny themselves nourishment through crash dieting also lack the energy to cope with a working day, and are equally vulnerable to an attack of Black Dog. It's that principle of balance, once again, which cannot be over-emphasised.

GETTING THE SUPPORT OF YOUR FAMILY

Before you embark on an exercise programme you must bring your weight under control by adopting healthy eating habits. If you live with a partner and/or children, their cooperation will be vitally important. No, don't say 'It can't be done, they won't change.'

Think of it this way. The improvement in your vitality will enhance the happiness of your family. Think of it as a gift from you to them. Remember, every coin has two sides – haven't you noticed? Each person in a relationship has an obligation to help the other. That's the life deal. The deal is that in enjoying the benefits of living and working together we have to help each other. Your partner and children will benefit from your success in taming your Black Dog and they have a responsibility to help you. If they can't see it, just tell them Patrick said so. *(See Chapter 16.)*

WHAT ABOUT DIETING?

I am suspicious of diets because they tend to be anti-social and call for a measure of willpower, which someone suffering from depression rarely has. Having said that, I managed, with excruciating determination, to diet seriously twice a year because as soon as I exceeded twelve-and-a-half stone my blood pressure soared. It was very sobering. These bi-annual diets had a seriously debilitating effect on me; the duration of my Black Dog attacks tended to lengthen and so did my drinking. Twice a year I took off over a stone in weight. Twice a year I was seriously depressed and twice a year I put more weight back on than I had taken off and was depressed again.

Many diets reduce both the calorie intake and nourishment. The result is you having neither adequate energy for a working day nor the resources to cope with the Black Dog. Furthermore, because your body is being denied adequate nourishment it goes on starvation alert. In this mode, when eventually you give yourself a square meal the body, instead of utilising the food to provide energy, puts it straight into store in the form of more fat to cater for the famine which your diet has told your body exists.

Eventually I discovered a meal replacement programme used by athletes, which together with pre-planned menus helped me to bring my weight permanently under control and provide me with the energy I needed.

INCREASED ENERGY LEVELS

Appropriate energy levels have an immediate and positive effect on our lifestyle. When we know we can do things without physical constraints we become more interested in everything that is happening around us. Because of this we start to do interesting things and spend time with interesting people. Because of our interest in life our morale improves, resulting in the Black Dog being squeezed out. We become, once more, a cheerful, helpful and effective person and as such a more interesting person to be with. Our self-esteem starts to reassert itself.

GETTING ENOUGH SLEEP

Adequate sleep is an essential component of energy. It is the way we recharge our banks of batteries. One battery is concerned with the cellular structure of our bodies, another provides energy for our emotions, another for our nervous system, and yet another for our mental processes.

> *Sleeplessness saps our vitality. It is a feature and symptom of depression and it is ruinous.*

Without a proper night's sleep we cannot function properly. We wander round with a whirly bird in our head and are subject to the most severe Black Dog attacks. This is a real problem because we cannot cure it until the causes have been eradicated and that, by their very nature, can take time. However, while you are dealing with your threatening life problems and the associated assaults of the Black Dog you will find that medication can be of enormous help.

While I was struggling with the impact of an unwanted divorce and the threat of financial calamity as well as the enthusiastic attentions of my Black Dog, my doctor prescribed a light sleeping aid, which helped me through a particularly bad six months. As my nourishment and exercise programmes kicked in and the demoralising unhappiness associated with the divorce procedures resolved itself, I naturally discontinued them. It just sort of happened. So supervised medication is a good idea if you are experiencing prolonged insomnia. (See Appendix 1.)

GETTING STARTED

Your objective, my friend, is to **increase your vitality by nourishment, exercise and rest.** And we'll start with nourishment.

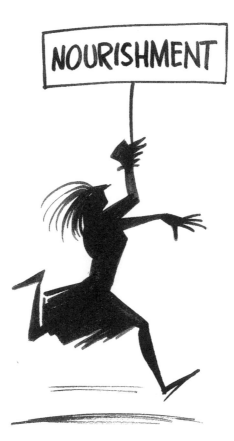

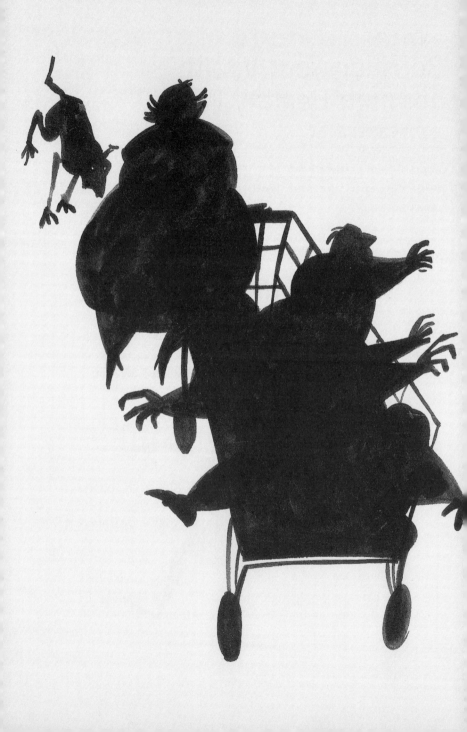

Chapter 11

Boosting Your Vitality Through Healthy Eating

YOU MIGHT BE WONDERING WHAT HEALTHY EATING has to do with taming the Black Dog. The answer is: we are what we eat.

The sort of food that we eat directly affects our propensity for depression.

The Black Dog thrives on chips, hamburgers, lots of bread, fatty meats, regular fry-ups, suet pastries, cakes, éclairs, sugary pies, toffees, sweet drinks and chocolate bars. It also loves snacks throughout the day. It will become the devoted companion of anyone regularly eating junk food and drinking too much alcohol.

These foods are high in sugar, starch, salt and fats. These are sources of immediate energy, which if not utilised by seriously heavy physical exertion, will be stored by the body as fat. This process is a rapid one and it is cumulative. The more fat you accumulate the less energy you have, the heavier you become and the more energy you need simply to move your body from A to B. Left alone it is a self-destruct mechanism.

Every time I shop at the supermarket I am appalled to see obese men and women, waddling round, often accompanied by overweight children, pushing a trolley piled high with hundreds of pounds' worth of what for the main part is junk food, with not a spring onion in sight, and a salivating Black Dog slinking just behind them.

They are what I call negative foods, because by themselves they have a negative influence on our health. So you'd better stop here for a moment to consider your present eating habits and decide whether the cap fits. OK?

EATING FOR BALANCE AND ENERGY

Your nourishment, like everything else, has to be kept in balance if you are to obtain the energy you need to lead an active, interesting and useful life. So what are we looking for? Why – surprise, surprise – we are looking for positive foods. And what are positive foods?

They include all the fresh foods. Green salads, most vegetables, including onions and leeks, and all the fruits. Fish, game and chicken cooked in olive oil and served hot or cold. These foods provide all the vitamins, minerals and trace elements you need to keep the cellular structure of your body healthy and your immune system effective. They are light on calories and therefore are useful in helping to burn up the fat that self-indulgent eating has created. If you live a physically demanding life you need some carbohydrates as well for short-term energy. In short, you need a balanced diet to lead a balanced and useful life.

MEAL REPLACEMENT NUTRITION PROGRAMMES

But if you are seriously overweight – five or six stones or more – how do you break the cycle of dieting and putting the weight back on?

I searched for years looking for a nourishment programme which, whilst restricting my tendency to accumulate fat, would provide energy. I needed the vitality to cope with the stresses and vicissitudes of my life at the time and to handle the Black Dog. I decided to investigate how athletes and astronauts approached this problem and came across the idea of measured and balanced nutrition taken in drink and tablet form for two meals each day, the third being a normal social meal shared with the family.

I decided to try it. Anything, but anything, I thought, would have to be an improvement on my twice-yearly crash diet followed by the long-term increase in my average weight and the associated depressions. I discovered a range of products, which were supplied under continuing supervision by a consultant, with nourishment programmes devised specially for an individual's needs. One programme, for example, was devised for people convalescing from surgery, another for athletes, others specially devised for men and women of particular age groups and another – the one that I was seeking – for active men and women who have a weight problem.

I did precisely what I was told to do and lost two stones in two months while experiencing increasing vigour and without the Black Dog. Because my body was receiving all the nutrients, vitamins, minerals and trace elements it needed it did not go onto starvation alert as it did when I was crash-dieting. The result was that during an indulgent holiday in France I only put on three or four pounds and had discarded them within a fortnight of returning.

I also found that for me it had two other hidden benefits. First, it was quick to prepare and during the day could be supplemented by muesli, yoghurt and dried and fresh fruit, which was great for someone with a demanding lifestyle and living on their own. The second was that I love food and enjoy cooking so I was able to have a good evening meal comprising fresh meat, chicken, game or fish, vegetables, sometimes fresh brown bread and butter or potatoes, but never both, and half a bottle of wine or a couple of cans of dry cider. My social life was unaffected because I could entertain and enjoy being entertained at dinner parties without fussing overly about what was being served.

After two years this programme is now a permanent feature of my life and I place my orders each month as part of my grocery purchases. So the cost comes out of my household budget.

There are three international companies whose naturally sourced products are approved by the governments of the UK, USA and most EU countries. One company provides a medical advisory service for GPs and also advises the American Olympics committee and netball association on nutritional programmes for athletes. See Appendix 2.

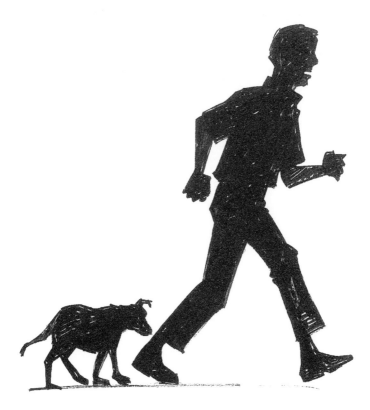

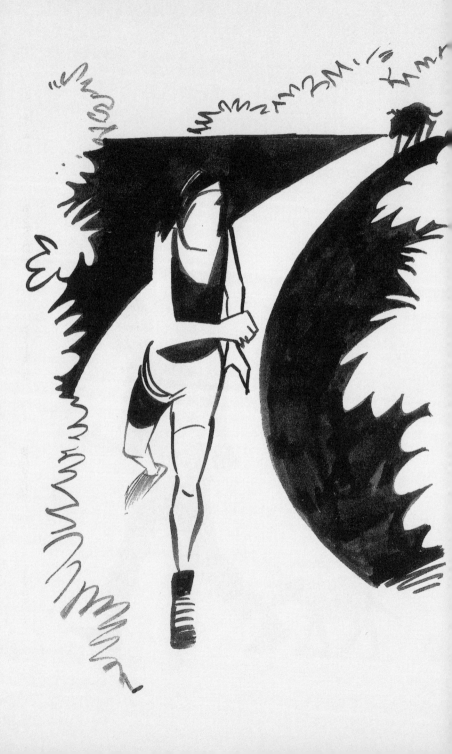

Chapter 12

Boosting Your Vitality Through Exercise

EXERCISE IS A KEY WAY OF PROVIDING ENERGY to tame the Black Dog.

The following exercise programme will improve your physical fitness; it will freshen up your mind every time you do it, and relax you. Combined with a 20-minute brisk walk or run, plus good nourishment, it will help to increase your capacity to cheerfully handle the vicissitudes of daily life and rise above the debilitating effects of depression.

WHY DO THESE EXERCISES?

The exercises offer many benefits:

- Immediate physical and mental well-being each morning.
- They only take 20 minutes. Not a moment longer.
- No equipment is needed.
- There is no need to join a gym.
- When you travel you can take them with you.
- They prepare your muscles for sporting activities.
- They are safe.

Quite quickly each day you will experience a feeling of enhanced well-being and you will develop the moral stamina to rise above the morning wave of assaults from the Black Dog.

Walk briskly to the station, take the stairs rather than the lift and you have completed a full 40-minute exercise regime each day.

It doesn't matter where you are. If you travel abroad on business as I do, you can do them in your hotel room. All that is needed is sufficient space for you to lie down, extend you arms above you and to each side and to swing round from the waist.

You do not need a gymnasium or fancy equipment like a rowing machine or static bicycle to get yourself fit. Indeed, in my experience most people are better off without these pieces of equipment. They tend to develop only one part of the muscle structure, leaving some groups weak and in danger of being wrenched, which can lead to skeletal problems.

This programme is safe and well proven and is based on the exercise regime practised by British, Canadian and American armed forces personnel in sedentary occupations. They are devised to achieve fitness and suppleness appropriate to one's age. They prepare the various muscle groups to undertake physical exertion such as walking, riding, skiing, jogging or other sports.

There is also an added value for people of more mature years. Back and joint pains often diminish and even disappear as your muscle groups strengthen and become pliable again.

DO'S AND DON'TS

Although these exercises are suitable for people of virtually every age group, you should advise your doctor of what you intend to do if you are receiving medication for blood pressure, or any heart, circulatory or respiratory complaint, or if you have any injuries.

1. Always occupy the full 20 minutes, not by doing more than is recommended in each table, but by doing each exercise slowly and as near perfectly as you can. I recommend that you exercise in front of a full-length mirror, particularly during the first month when you will be aiming for perfection and suppleness rather than increased exertion. (You can stick your foundation habits and daily positive commitment habits on it – *see Chapters 6 and 7*. Once you are familiar with the exercises you can recite your daily commitments at the same time.)

2. If you experience joint or muscle pain when you promote yourself to the next table, immediately revert to the previous table again for another three days. Suffering is not a part of this programme.

3. Continuity is vital. Lack of continuity will damage both muscle and mind. However, allow yourself one day off each week. The weekends are best for the rest day.

4. A hot shower or quick hot bath and rub down afterwards will set you up for the day. By all means have a cold one as well. It really stimulates body and mind. However, I must confess to having given the cold one up some years ago. But, hell, I'm older than you, so get under it!

5. This is not a muscle-building programme. It is a fitness creation programme which will permit you to play competitive sports like tennis, squash, fencing, badminton, netball or football safely, or to start to enjoy jogging, riding, skiing or even bungie jumping if you are that way inclined (something I hasten to add that I am not recommending!). It will also improve your golf.

> ### When's the best time to exercise?
> *Do the exercises and walk or run before breakfast. Why? To get out of the house as quickly as possible in order to escape the almost inevitable Black Dog dawn patrol. The exception to this is if on the way to work you are incorporating a two-mile walk to the station as part of your daily programme. It's important not to skip breakfast* (see Chapter 11).

THE MUSCLE GROUPS

There are ten groups of muscles that we are going to make equally strong and pliable:

1. Neck muscles.
2. Shoulder and shoulder blade muscles.
3. Chest expansion muscles.
4. Waist muscles back and front.
5. Waist muscles sideways.
6. Back and twist muscles.
7. Thigh muscles.
8. Stomach muscles.
9. Leg muscles.
10. Back muscles.

In addition we will stretch the whole frame and correct the posture.

THE EFFECTS ON YOUR LIFE

Physical well-being will improve your posture and therefore your body language. It is probable that unknowingly you have developed a body language that reflects your depressed mental outlook. These exercises will not only correct this handicap physically but will bolster your mental attitude as well. The hang-dog posture manifested by many depressives during an attack will disappear. The round-shouldered slouch will be replaced with a head-up and erect positive posture. When explaining or discussing something with business colleagues or friends your body will exude energy and enthusiasm for what you are saying. The enhanced optimism will help you to become more tolerant and therefore improve your relationships. Your whole demeanour will become more positive and it will become easier for other people to interact with you in a more creative way.

Just as mind influences matter, so physical well-being improves your attitude. The body is the temple of the soul and to develop mentally and spiritually you need a healthy body.

Please do not be tempted to defeat this truism by producing examples of people with devastated bodies who exude unbelievable cheerfulness in adversity and magnificent courage in suffering, as well as a unique level of ability, like Stephen Hawkins. They are the exceptions and we should make use of their example to master our own relatively meagre affliction.

YOUR EXERCISE PROGRAMME

For absolute beginners up to 70 years old.

Each exercise to be done only three times for the first week or until you are executing each one perfectly in front of the mirror slowly and smoothly and without aches or pains. Be gentle with yourself. Use the 10 x 12 fitness programme on page 106 to record your progress.

Group 1 – neck muscles

1. Stand erect in front of the mirror. Place feet about two feet apart and put hands on waist. Push out your chin as far as possible and hold it for a moment. Now draw back your head and tuck in your chin. Hold for a moment and relax. Now repeat the exercise three times.

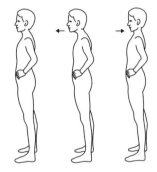

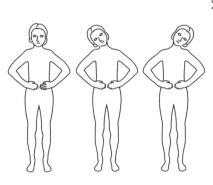

2. Drop your head sideways onto your left shoulder and hold for a moment. Now bring it back and let it fall onto your right shoulder and hold for a moment. Repeat three times slowly and then relax your neck muscles with your head in the upright position.

3. Drop your head forwards so that your chin rests on your chest and you are looking at the floor and hold for a moment. Now slowly bring your head through the upright and let it fall back so that you are looking upwards at the ceiling. Repeat three times and relax.

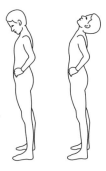

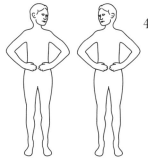

4. In the upright position, turn your head to the left until you are looking over your left shoulder and pause. Now slowly turn your head until you are looking directly over your right shoulder and pause. Repeat three times, then relax looking directly forward.

5. The next exercise is head rolling and older people should have a support of some kind, like the back of a chair, close by in case they become dizzy. It is a combination of the previous exercises executed in one smooth movement through a complete circle. Roll three times one way without stopping and thee times in the opposite direction. On completion of the exercise do what ballet dancers do, turn your head quickly and once in the opposite direction to maintain your inner ear balance. Finish looking directly ahead, take a deep breath and relax.

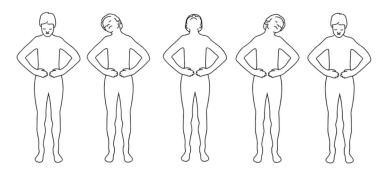

Group 2 – chest expansion and shoulder muscles

1. With you hands still on your waist, push your shoulders up into a shrug then rotate them forward and downwards. At the lowest point start to press them back and up whilst continuing the rotary movement and regaining the shrug. Repeat three times smoothly and relax. Now do the exercise again in the reverse direction rotating your shoulders from the shrug backwards in a rotary action. Repeat three times. Take a deep breath, exhale and relax.

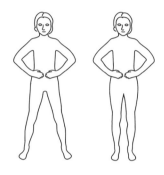

2. Extend your arms sideways and hold for a moment. Now bending your arms at the elbow, fold your forearms forward with your palms towards the ground, then bring them round towards you until your forefingers touch your chest at shoulder height. Press shoulders back three times, then throw your arms wide open and backwards at shoulder level. Drop arms by side. Repeat the whole exercise thee times.

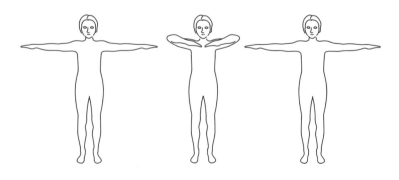

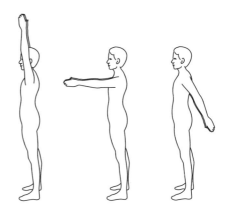

3. Stretch your arms vertically above you and reach for the ceiling. Now rotate them forwards trying to make them brush your ears at the top of the swing and brushing your hips at the bottom of the rotation. Do it smoothly three times and relax. Now repeat in the reverse direction three times. Take a deep breath, exhale and relax.

Group 3 – waist muscles

There are four exercises for this group: bending forwards and back; bending side to side; swinging above the hips; and the windmill.

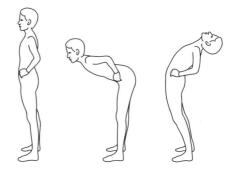

1. Face the mirror, feet apart with your hands on your waist. Take a deep breath. Now continuing to look at your face in the mirror slowly bend forward from the hips and exhale at the same time. Keep your back hollow and do not allow either your back or shoulders to become rounded. Go down as far as you can, keeping your legs straight. Pause for a moment. Now breathing in slowly, return through the erect position until you are leaning as far

back as you can without toppling over or straining, exhaling again at the same time. Let your head fall back until you are looking at the ceiling and hold it for a moment. Return through the erect position until you are leaning forward again, at the same time breathing in and then exhaling on the way down. Repeat three times.

2. Start with feet apart and hands on waist. Look over your left shoulder and slowly lean over sideways from the waist, at the same time looking down the side of your legs. Push and hold, then return through the erect position. Looking over the 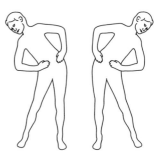 right shoulder, go down as far as you can on the right side. Hold it, then repeat smoothly and slowly three times.

3. With feet apart, extend your arms sideways at shoulder height. Holding your hips still, swing your arms round to the left whilst looking as far left as you can. Immediately swing back as far right as you can. Put plenty of energy into the swinging action so that your arms will pull your trunk round and stretch the muscles.

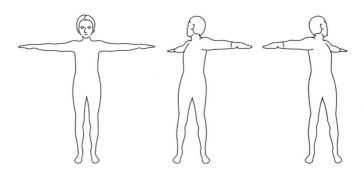

4. The windmill is the combination of the three previous exercises in one continuous rotating motion. As usual start with your feet well apart. Look up at the ceiling and stretch your arms up as though you were going to touch it. Twist your trunk to the left and look left. Slowly swing left and downwards, bending your whole body and with straight legs try to brush the floor with your hands. Continue the rotation, twisting and looking to the right as you windmill upwards and back to the starting position. Don't stop, continue with the windmilling slowly and smoothly for three rotations. Relax, take a deep breath, exhale and repeat the exercise starting with the right swing. Repeat three times then deep breath, exhale and relax.

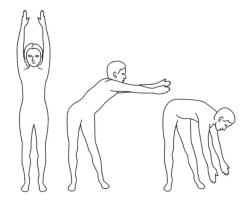

Group 4 – thighs, knee bends, waist twisting

This can be a difficult exercise for older people who are unaccustomed to exercise. But don't be discouraged – eventually you will be able to do it. It's a great exercise for once-a-year skiers. Initially you may need some support while regaining your balance and developing the strength in your thigh and calf muscles. Hold onto the rim of a pedestal wash basin, a radiator or a chair.

1. Stand to attention with feet together and hands on waist. Go onto the balls of your feet by raising your heels. Looking steadily ahead at a fixed point, slowly bend the knees and go down until you are sitting on your heels in a full knees-bend position. Give a little bounce 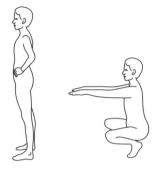 then straighten your legs, rising to the tip-toe position, and slowly lower your heels onto the ground. Repeat this three times.

2. Sit cross legged on the floor or as near to cross legged as you can without falling over. Stretch out your arms sideways at shoulder height. Swing your arms round to the left looking as far to the left as you can then swing to the right looking as far to the right as you can. Repeat this three times.

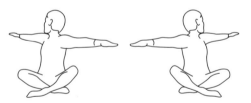

Group 5 – stretching abdominal muscles and correcting posture

1. Lie on your back on the floor, legs together and arms by your side with the palms of your hands facing downwards. Lie perfectly straight and make yourself comfortable by adjusting your head and neck, trunk and legs. Now slowly take a deep

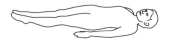

breath and when you feel your lungs are full try to take in more air. Go on, more, more, more… hold it for three or four seconds. Let it go. Force every drop of air out until your lungs are empty. Slowly let them fill to normal and relax. Repeat three times. A word of warning: some people who are doing deep breathing for the first time may experience a slight feeling of dizziness. This is because your body is unused to handling so much oxygen. It is called hyper-ventilation. Just rest and breath shallowly and normally for a minute and it will quickly disappear. Then resume the exercise.

2. Still lying on the floor, bend your left leg at the knee, bringing the heel backwards until it is touching your buttock. Holding this leg position, lift your right hand keeping the arm straight, rotate it backwards and try to make the back of your hand touch the floor over your head. Many people will be unable to do this at first, but as the muscle groups stretch and your spine straightens the back of the hand will get closer and closer to the floor until after your third week you should be able to achieve it with little difficulty. It gets easier and easier. Straighten your leg and bring your arm to your side, palm down again. Now do the same with your right leg and left arm. Relax. Repeat the whole exercise three times.

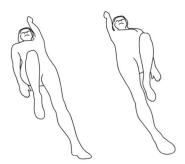

Group 6 – abdominal muscles and neck

1. Lie on your back on the floor. Bend both legs at the knee with the feet drawn towards you. Place your hands palms down on your thighs. Now focussing your eyes on the top of your knees, lift your shoulders off the floor and try to touch your knees with your fingers. Hold for a moment and then lie back and relax. You may not be able to make your fingers touch your knees at first but you will feel your tummy muscles contracting and straining. You will find that as you persevere your shoulders will come further off the floor, which means that your tummy muscles are strengthening and tightening.

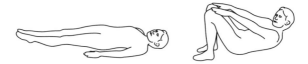

2. Lie perfectly straight on your back with legs outstretched and arms beside you palms down. Lift the left leg until it is vertical and as near straight as you can make it. Slowly lower it towards the ground, stopping for three seconds when your heel is an inch or two from the floor, then continue to lower it and relax. Do the same with your right leg and repeat the whole exercise three times. Relax. Later, when your tummy muscles have strengthened, lift both legs together.

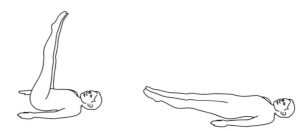

Group 7 – thigh, hip and waist muscles

Lie on your left side with your head supported on your bent left arm and hand. Look down your body towards your feet and adjust your position until your body is perfectly straight. Now keeping your right leg straight, lift it up as far as it will go. Hold it for a moment and slowly return it to lie on top of the other. Repeat three times. Turn onto your right side and repeat the exercise three times. Relax.

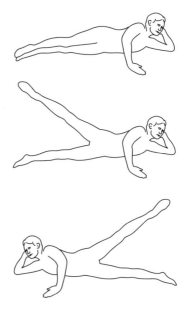

Group 8 – back and spinal muscles

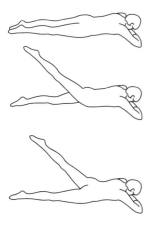

1. Lie on your tummy with your arms folded above your head and your forehead resting on the back of your hands. Try to lift your right leg off the floor, keeping it straight, until you feel your thigh come off the floor. You will also feel your big back muscles start to pull. Hold it for a moment, then lower to the floor. Do the same with your left leg. Now repeat the whole exercise three times and relax.

2. Continue to lie on your tummy and place your hands palms upwards under your thighs. Lift both legs and head, hold for two seconds and relax. Initially the movement will be small but as your back muscles strengthen you will be able to lift your legs higher.

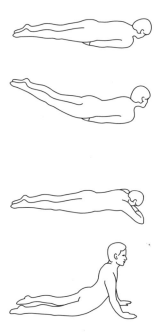

3. Continue to lie on your tummy but place your hands under your chest and push up, straightening your arms. This will curve your spine and start to strengthen your shoulder muscles. Hold it and lower yourself to the floor. Repeat three times.

Group 9 – Rolling Ball – Spine Strengthening

Make yourself into a ball by adopting a little girl sitting position with your knees snuggled into your chest and your arms hugging your legs and holding them tightly into you. Your back will be rounded and so will your shoulders. Now, hugging yourself tightly, push yourself backwards with your toes and roll onto your back until your trunk is above your head and your neck is being bent. Using your head and neck muscles, give a push so that you roll forwards into a sitting position again and immediately roll back again. Repeat this three times, getting

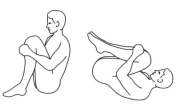

a good active backwards and forwards rolling motion. If at first you have difficulty in rolling forward again, then straighten your legs a little, using them as a counterbalance.

Group 10 – Balance

This last exercise will improve your balance. Some older people may find that balance eludes them at first but persevere because it will strengthen your confidence in your own agility and will permit you to put your pants on with a degree of elegance without falling about the bedroom.

Stand erect and relaxed in front of your full length mirror. Now whilst focussing on the reflection of your eyes in the mirror, slowly lift your left knee, and as it comes up to your waist height, clasp it and pull it in to your chest. Then lower it. Regain your balance and repeat with the right leg. Try to do the whole exercise smoothly as though you were doing a slow march on the spot.

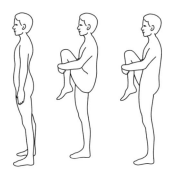

Group 11 – Running on the spot
Start with 100 paces and record the time it takes.

Run on your toes and lift your knees as high as you can. You will quickly find that your pulse speeds up and your breathing speeds up and gets deeper. At the end you should have started to sweat. You count each pace when your left foot touches the ground. Every three days increase the number of paces you record by five.

10 by 12 Fitness Programme

Muscle group	Exercise number	Time allotted (seconds)	Wk1 2 3	Wk2 4	Wk3 5 6	Wk4 7	Wk5 8	Wk6 9	Wk7 10	Wk8 11	Wk9 12	Wk10 12	Wk11 12	Wk12 12	Wk13 13	Wk14 14	Wk15 15	Wk16 16
							Number of repeats per three day and six day periods											
I	1	20																
	2	20																
	3	20																
	4	20																
	5	20																
II	1	20																
	2	20																
	3	20																
III	1	30																
	2	30																
	3	30																
	4	50																
IV	1	30																
	2	30																
V	1	60																
	2	30																
VI	1	30																
	2	30																
VII	1	30																
	2	30																
VIII	1	30																
	2	30																
	3	30																
IX	1	50																
X	1	30																

Finally

Take a 20-minute brisk walk or do five minutes' running on the spot (see below) and you will have tamed the Black Dog and be ready to manage your day. You just see. To finish off have a hot shower or bath, followed by a cold douche if you are brave enough. Have a cup of tea and a good breakfast *(see Chapter 11).*

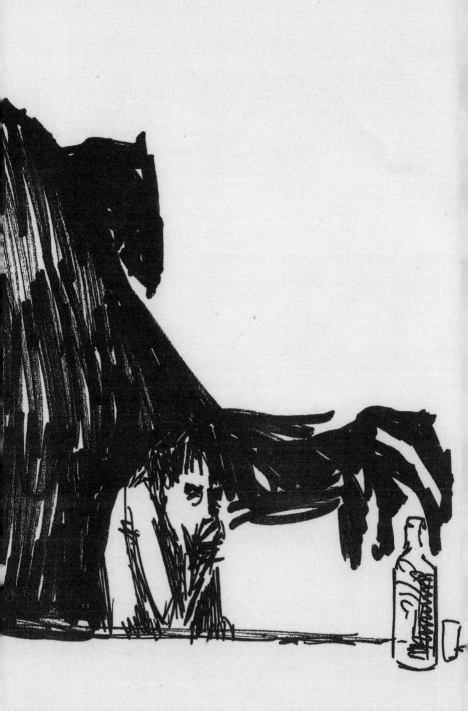

Chapter 13
Alcohol Management

THE CONSUMPTION OF ALCOHOL IS AN INTEGRAL PART of most people's social life. It can enhance our enjoyment of events, enliven our contribution to the fun of others and relax the nature of our relationships, for a short time, provided – and always provided – it is taken in moderation.

The old adage says that alcohol is a good friend but a bad enemy. For the depressive, alcohol is a poison. Got it?

Alcohol is a poison.

Quantities of alcohol that would be considered moderate for many people are poisonous to a depressive. The Black Dog thrives on the aftermath of its influence and its attacks can be devastating.

Relax – I am not going to advise you to abstain from drinking altogether, although you ought to while you are taking prescribed medication. I am insisting that you consider the consequences of drinking even a small amount too much. I am insisting that you plan your consumption of alcohol, and manage it when you are socialising. It can be done and the benefit in terms of morale and restful sleep is almost immediate.

THE EFFECTS OF ALCOHOL

First let us consider why alcohol is a poison, how it becomes poisonous and what its effects are on our ability to lead a normal life.

Many depressives, if not all who drink, do so unwittingly for medicinal purposes. We have a shot in the arm to overcome our low self-esteem. It gives us a lift and diminishes self-doubt. Our social confidence is strengthened and we feel that we are in control of ourselves and our lives. It's a great feeling to be relieved from the servitude of despair.

This is the first drink. The sugar provides short-term energy and the alcohol dilates our arteries. The brain is stimulated by the increased blood flow and so are our muscles, promoting a feeling of vitality and optimism. We've really knocked the Black Dog on the head, ha, ha, ha.

With the second drink we feel normal and free of inhibitions. Life is just as it should be – gorgeous – and so are we. In fact, our critical faculties are already being dulled, and we can become as high with the elation of alcohol as previously we were diminished by depression. When someone suggests another bottle of wine or another round of drinks we are surprised that they have been so reticent. Of course it goes without saying that we should have another one. For goodness sake, who could have thought otherwise?

The third drink relaxes us completely and we tend to become a bit sentimental or, paradoxically, bellicose. The depressive effect of alcohol insinuates its way into our system. The joie de vivre is not as keen as it was an hour ago. So we think another drink will do no harm; indeed it's rather a good idea. It will just put us on top again. Back in control!

This is an ephemeral illusion, which evaporates as soon as our head hits the pillow and even before then if the drink has made us argumentative. This is a time when other people's sensitivities can be affronted. But the worst is yet to come.

After three or four hours we are wakened by the call of nature and emerge into a hell on earth. Much more than a hangover, far worse. To make matters worse, this awakening coincides with the lowest time for our metabolism. The Black Dog has us on the floor. In the darkness in our remorseful state we see ourselves as we think others saw us – and particularly our loved ones – a foolish exhibitionist compensating for his or her own inadequacy. Our diminished opinion of ourselves is reinforced. Tasks that need attention in the morning assume threatening and impossible proportions. The certain knowledge that we cannot cope with the coming day drives us down still further. Fear, unmitigated and stark, comes out of its box and we curl up in a foetal ball – paralysed.

If we are alone in bed we writhe and toss and whimper as the Black Dog savages us. If our partner is by our side we grit our teeth and stiffen so as not to wake them. We are consumed by a pain, as physical as it is emotional. Every atom of our being cries out for relief from the choking despondency and even suicide seems a desirable option.

Eventually light creeps through the curtains and fearfully we crawl out of bed to attend to our ablutions. We look down onto the outside world and see real people and birds and cars going about their business. In a sort of grey aching haze we go down to make a cup of tea or coffee and slowly emerge into the reality of the day, like a soldier coming out of his dugout after enduring a night of bombardment, bemused and shaken.

We get ourselves to work, weary and purposeless, and our colleagues laughingly and some not so laughingly comment that we are not as perky as usual and conclude that we've had a row at home or a good party.

Such a scenario can be and often is brought about by just one glass of wine too many, or that last pint of beer. The results are not just painful but for the depressive they are downright dangerous. Therefore, for safety's sake, we must have a plan of alcohol management which we practise every day as part of our positive habit commitments.

If you think you can stop drinking alcohol altogether until you have tamed your Black Dog completely, do so.

YOUR ALCOHOL PLAN

1. Consult your daily diary *(see Chapter 4)* and see how much alcohol you are consuming and where and when.

2. Consider an alternative way of occupying yourself instead of drinking, and do it.

3. Construct a daily habit commitment to overcome your alcohol habit and repeat it six times morning and evening.

I .... sleep restfully without alcohol.
*I .... choose not to drink during the week
and feel really good.*

4. Visualise how awful you feel after drinking too much. Bring
   up the memory of the emotions and physical sensations you
   experience and the demoralisation of the Black Dog attack.
   Focus on it, re-live every second of it, until you are almost
   experiencing the symptoms again. Practise doing this until
   you can call up the sensation and sense of demoralisation at
   will. Whenever you want a drink or when you are offered a
   drink, call up this atrocious memory and concentrate on it.
   Now decide how best to avoid it.

5. Plan how much (if any) alcohol you are going to consume
   each day. Each morning repeat your alcohol management
   plan for the day, six times.

   *Tonight I will drink two glasses of water when I arrive home and one
   glass of wine or cider with my meal. I really no longer need alcohol.*

   *Tonight I am meeting Jack for a drink. I will have two half pints of
   cider or beer. No more.*

   I do not need alcohol. I am the general commanding my life.

6. Drink two glasses of water every hour throughout the day.
   This will prevent you becoming dehydrated and stop you
   drinking alcohol to quench your thirst.

7. Never drink alcohol at lunchtime. There is no compromise here.

8. When you are attending a dinner party drink at least one glass of water with each glass of wine. It is no use waiting until you are about to leave for a dinner party and saying I'll only have three glasses of wine tonight. After the third glass you will have forgotten whether you had the first and in all probability overlooked the gin and tonic beforehand.

9. Alcohol management must be practised as a daily commitment until it becomes an established positive habit and you have assumed control of your life.

10. Enlist the help of your partner or a friend. We all need help and encouragement. Very few can do it on their own.

11. Talk with your mentor *(see Chapter 14)*.

When implemented as an integral part of the programme for taming the Black Dog, managing your alcohol consumption is less difficult than you might imagine.

SUMMARY

■ Alcohol is a poison, especially for someone who is prone to depression.

■ Reduce your alcohol consumption to a level that does not adversely affect you.

■ Plan how much you are going to drink each day.

■ Include alcohol management in your auto-suggestion routine.

■ Never drink alcohol at lunchtime.

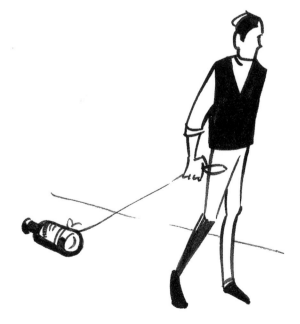

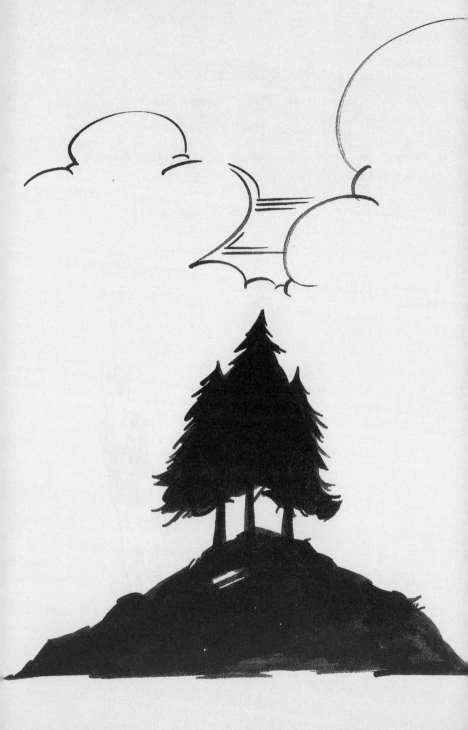

Chapter 14
Finding a Mentor

EVERYONE NEEDS A MENTOR TO GUIDE THEM and to help them to set appropriate criteria against which to measure their performance and behaviour. Our first mentors are our parents – or should be.

In adult life many people seem not to have a mentor, and therefore measure their standards of behaviour and performance against that of their peers. Here we have an expanding social problem. We all know that just trying to keep up with someone else is impossible because we always fall behind by a small amount. We only take in about 60 per cent of what we say to each other. This means that if maintaining acceptable standards of behaviour in our society relies on peer criteria, then our society is in a progressive state of deterioration!

We need to admire a mentor and he or she needs to be in some respects superior to ourselves in order to provide informed counselling. Their strengths should counteract our own weaknesses. Being able to appreciate another person's achievements and superiority in some measure is not to diminish ourselves. Indeed it is a sign of our own maturity.

We need different mentors at different times in our lives. Our parents, a schoolteacher, a superior officer, tutor, boss or an admired friend. These are the people to whom we go for guidance and help, who help us to find a purpose in life, and most importantly encourage us to drive forward towards high achievement.

Every successful person has or has had a mentor, who sets them high criteria for performance and attainment. Top opera singers and musicians all have mentors who are their teachers. Top Olympic riders have riding masters and Winston Churchill had Clementine. So who is your mentor?

CHOOSING YOUR MENTOR

He or she will surely be someone who respects and admires you, as you respect and admire them. They will be competent to advise you, wise, approachable, honest, understanding, patient and without malice. A lot to ask for, you might think. Not really, providing you share mutual affection and you respect their superior knowledge. How to elicit their help? Why, ask them, of course. People are usually glad to help someone in difficulties. They, too, derive fulfilment and a sense of reward from helping someone along life's road.

Just one important thing. It's a good idea to know how and why you want them to be your mentor before trotting round to see them. You must be ready to be candid in sharing your difficulties with them and have decided on the sort of help you need. If you need help in coping with your depression, be open about it. You have nothing to be ashamed of. Talk about it in terms of your aspirations and expectations. So go get a mentor, and good luck!

A DIFFERENT KIND OF MENTOR

Note to readers: Because this book is autobiographical, this chapter touches on the role of God as my mentor. Those of you who follow a faith other than Christianity will have your own role model, your own God to whom you can turn. Don't hesitate, use your faith. Those of you who are clever enough to be atheistic can skip this next bit. If you are an agnostic I would advise you to keep your options open and to read on. It just might be a posh word for ignorance in your case.

Without a mentor we can become disorientated and vulnerable. I know. At a time in my life when I desperately needed one there was nobody to turn to. My parents were dead, so was my old commanding officer, and I was afraid of confiding my difficulties to my wife. I was head of my own business so I had no boss or superior to talk to and I didn't think that my bank manager had the necessary qualifications. To make matters worse, the Black Dog was magnifying my problems and so was alcohol.

I desperately needed someone to turn to and it was only then that very slowly it began to dawn on me that in truth I had always had a mentor who had been watching me all my life. I did not have his telephone number but I thought that I knew how to get in touch with him and I knew his name. It is Jesus.

Oh dear, I hear you murmur, not another religious crank. Not at all. In fact a very practically minded person who has experienced the impact of the Black Dog in moments of outstanding achievement and devastating failure and who has explored many avenues to defeat it. This is one of those avenues and you will find it interacts comfortably with the other methods in this book.

Over the years my spiritual relationship with God had been weakened by my own intellectual arrogance and obscured by poorly conceived sermons preached by priests of the established churches who were out of touch with the reality of my own contemporary life. I had started to deny the evidence of my own spirituality, a common cause of depression. My parents had made him the prime motivator in their lives, so I asked myself why he should not motivate me as well.

As these thoughts began to take shape I realised that I was contemplating the greatest role model, who 2000 years ago galvanised the world when he introduced the concept of love being central to everything and in so doing released the most dynamic creative power the world has ever known. Here was the world's greatest philosopher, whose teachings embrace the positive and loving aspects of other faiths and who was available to me if I wanted him. Exciting stuff, eh?

I decided, for the time being at any rate, to separate my concept of him from the difficult and confusing theological ideas of a life hereafter and the resurrection of the body. I focussed on Jesus himself as a teacher and as my prospective mentor now.

What did I unearth that was relevant to me? I realised that he was a wholly positive person who taught that the power of love is the central ingredient in dealing with the problems of our lives and the nature of our relationships. He replaced the established negative teachings starting with 'thou shalt not' with positive ones starting with operative verbs like '**love** thy neighbour,' '**come** to me,' '**go** into the world'. His focus is on the future and never on the past. Indeed, he deals with the past appropriately when he tells us that if we admit our sins – in modern parlance, our failures, bad decisions, cruelty and thoughtless behaviour – and ask for forgiveness from God, we will be forgiven. In other words, our failures and mistakes are a thing of the past so we don't have to waste our valuable time worrying about them. Most importantly I found that I could talk to him in complete honesty about my successes as well as my mistakes and receive his assurance of hope.

I found that I could share my confusion with him and ask him to help me find a way through troubled waters. And he did.

My purpose in revealing this particular aspect of my own life is that when I was lonely, isolated, diminished, with the Black Dog threatening me, I was able to take Jesus on board as my mentor and with him set fresh criteria and purpose for my future. This book is a result.

Everyone can make their God their mentor, whenever they choose.

Asking for inspiration and guidance

How on earth, or heaven for that matter, do I do that, I hear you ask. Well, you ask him, of course, just like anyone else you want help from. Describe to him your problems, share with him your worries and fears and ask him to give inspiration and guidance. Then be silent and let the thoughts moving around your mind slowly come to the surface. Get on with your work and plan your future. Before going to bed sit quietly and share your fears with him. Tell him your problems and ask him to inspire your thinking to find an answer. You do not ask him to solve your problems for you or to save you. You ask him for the inspiration for **you** to find a way of solving **your** difficulties. It's a dynamic form of meditation and it's called praying. Whoops!

Some years ago I had a friend who at the time was one of the country's leading psychiatrists. At the dinner table we were discussing whether religion or some belief in God had any relevance in modern day lives. He said, 'Patrick, if people knew how to pray my consulting couch would be mostly empty.'

You do not have to be religious or belong to a particular faith to pray for inspiration and to receive guidance. It is a simple God-given process, which works, although I don't know how. What I do know is that 'there are things in heaven and on earth, Horatio, that we know not of'.

Consider for a moment the forces of gravity, magnetism, electricity, radio and microwave transmission. They have existed since the start of the universe, just waiting for the ingenuity of man to work out how to harness them and turn them into sources of positive power. It is only in this last infinitesimal period of barely 200 years that their nature has been discovered. Consider the telepathic ability of animals and indeed our own and consider the effect that the moon and planets have on our climate, our emotions and our physiology. Is it beyond the bounds of probability that we humans do have unused receiving and transmitting capabilities, which are just waiting for us to develop? Dare we call this embryonic facility our spiritual being, and would it not be a wise thing to go in search of it?

There are huge extra-terrestrial influences at work over which as individuals we have neither understanding nor control. Supposing we visualise them collectively as comprising one universal eternal intelligence – what then? Having got so far, supposing we call this intelligence God. Not asking too much, is it? Not going beyond the bounds of credulity, are we?

So what happens if we address ourselves to him and ask for inspiration and guidance? Firstly we have to be dead honest. Because he is all-seeing we have to be truthful about our mistakes, failures and particularly about our successes.

There is no room for rationalisation or after-the-event wisdom. Most importantly there is no room for unnatural self-effacement and unsubstantiated self-criticism. Complete and uninhibited honesty about your achievements and feelings for others is necessary. In talking to your God, truthfully and factually, you will gain increasing self-knowledge, which in turn will help you find a purpose for your life, if you have not found one already. We begin to see ourselves as we really are, including our talents, and that's good. We have more to be proud of than to be ashamed of – lots more.

We have to be specific in our prayers, and the answer comes into our mind in the form of inspirational and creative thoughts. It is simply no use asking him to make our circumstances go away when we have contributed to them ourselves, nor to save us physically when we have placed ourselves in imminent danger.

If you jump out of an aeroplane crying 'God save me' without having taken the precaution of attaching yourself to a parachute, then you can be assured that Newton's Law of Gravity will prevail.

An inspirational speaker

Eric Jackson, a country preacher, had recovered from cancer through the power of prayer. He was not an ordained priest, but had the most profound effect on my understanding of God and where I stood in the scheme of things. I have to admit that at the time I was not there out of devotion. I happened to be playing the organ that Sunday and they couldn't start without me.

During his sermon – actually it was more a talk than a sermon – he looked out through the plain windows of our village church and pointed to what he called the wonder of God's kingdom manifested by the surrounding hills, the budding trees, the nesting birds, the emerging wheat and the young of every species and he said, 'There it is, the kingdom of God'. Then he looked at each one of us in the congregation and said, 'There you are, look at each other, there is the kingdom of God.' Then, after a moment or two of silence, his coup de grace: 'And the Kingdom of God is within each one of us. We humans are not outside God's kingdom. It is already within each one of us, and it's up to us whether we search for it, and how we utilise it.'

SUMMARY

- Everyone needs a mentor.

- One has different mentors at different times.

- Choose your mentor and ask for their help and advice – they will probably be flattered.

- Consider the possibility of your God as your mentor.

- Seek your own spirituality.

- Prayer is simply talking to your God.

- Ask for inspiration on how **you** can find a solution to your difficulties.

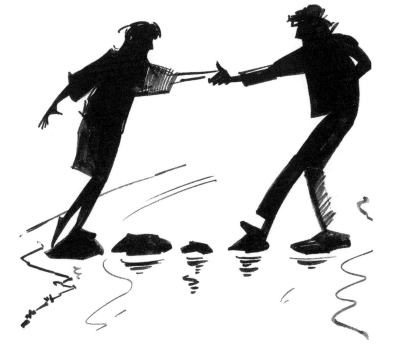

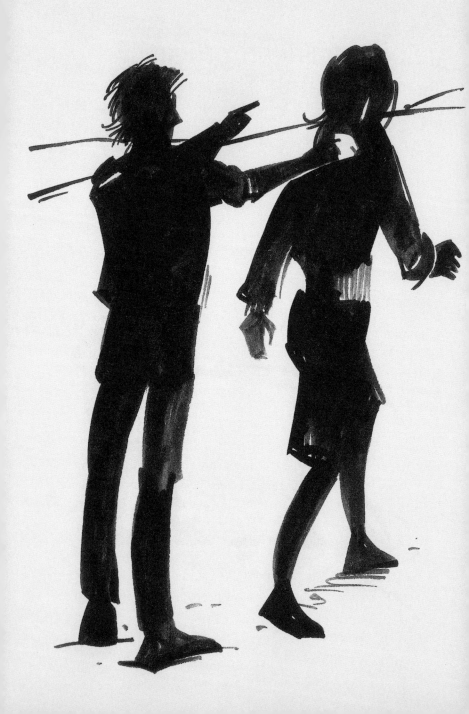

Chapter 15
Helping a Friend or Family Member Tame Their Black Dog

> *Depression is not just a state of mind. It affects a person's whole physiology. But helping someone to tame the Black Dog is not to nurse a sick person to health: it is to elevate a normal person to their full creative potential.*

LIVING WITH OR BEING CLOSE TO SOMEONE suffering from depression can be a test of one's affection. Fortunately, depression responds to medication, and to positive thinking therapy. Your support will be invaluable.

A NOTE ABOUT MANIC DEPRESSION

In my experience the most difficult depressive to help is the manic-depressive. While in the manic phase of their affliction their responses are over the top, to the point of their behaviour becoming bizarre. They often exude massive amounts of unfocussed mental energy and in this agitated state of mind believe that they are capable of achieving anything, which in certain inspired circumstances some of them do.

In this heightened state of mind they will not, perhaps cannot, respond to reasoned counselling from people close to them and refuse to accept that they need the calming effect of medication. They can become abusive and this makes it very difficult to maintain a constructive relationship with them. Even when you know that they are not their normal selves and that a usually considerate person is in the grip of an exceedingly wild and potentially dangerous member of the Black Dog breed, it can test one's patience and affection to breaking point. Under these circumstances you yourself must enlist professional guidance for both of you.

UNDERSTANDING DEPRESSION

You must accept that if you have never suffered from depression, you are unlikely to understand its effect on the outlook of the sufferer. During an attack of the Black Dog the fearful thoughts within a depressive's mind are more real to him or her than reality itself. At the time, these black thoughts will succumb to neither reason nor persuasion. You have to wait until they emerge into the light again before you can help. In the meantime, just remain friendly and adopt the role of a disinterested observer. Fortunately, in many cases Black Dog attacks – although repetitive – are like passing squalls in the climate of life. Make yourself familiar with their timings and with the procedures and exercises in this book.

WHAT TO DO

The first crucial step is to persuade the sufferer to consult his or her GP.

Care and sensitivity will be needed because for many people, particularly men, depression is a stigma. At the first mention of depression many men will react in a characteristically negative way. They will obstinately refuse to consider the possibility that they might be afflicted. They will repudiate it with the same irritation that they would if you suggested that they were alcohol dependant, which many will have become. The very idea questions their masculinity. They might have some or all of the following reactions:

Other people suffer from depression. People who suffer from it are nut cases. Damn it, I have a successful career.   What do you think people – my colleagues, my clients – would say if they thought I had depression? What would it do to my credibility? It brings into question my judgement. I resent your suggesting that I have this problem. It makes we wonder what you really think about me.

Women are less likely to react in such a vehement way, because they are usually more comfortable with problems of relationship and talk freely with each other on how best to solve them. They are usually more open-minded than the introspective male. However, all depressives have a propensity for irritability and even anger. It is a tricky business trying to help an angry person.

You may have to wait until an opportunity presents itself naturally. You might open the issue by mentioning casually that you saw an article on managing worry and stress and about people feeling down. Say that you had no idea how many people suffer from depression quite unnecessarily. One in ten people across the UK and as high as one in five businessmen and women. Musicians, writers, barristers, doctors, and politicians including, for example, Winston Churchill who suffered from it most of his life and called it the Black Dog.

Reflect aloud about the speed and pressure of contemporary life. Then remark that sometimes you feel affected yourself and have wondered whether to talk to your GP. If they show interest you can encourage the dialogue. If they back off, leave it for another day. The seed has been sown.

On the next suitable occasion remark that you have been feeling down and that you are considering getting a tonic or something from the doctor. After all, it would be silly not get some aspirin if you had a headache. Ask them for their opinion and advice.

Hopefully what was previously a private closed book will now open. A chat with the doctor, 'to get something to cheer us up', becomes an acceptable proposition. Encourage them gently, to help them to overcome their stubbornness and fear or their shyness and uncertainty.

> *The subterfuge is justified if it results in your partner or friend receiving appropriate medication and continuing professional supervision.*

If you attend the same doctors' surgery it is easy to bring the doctor on side at the outset. His or her involvement at the initial stage will be a tremendous benefit to both of you. I cannot over-emphasise the importance of communicating with your doctor. This book can then immediately start to play its role in damage repair. Your own resolve and encouragement will be invaluable. Just one further word of advice: keep your dialogue and relationship light-hearted and fun if you can. More about that later.

HELPING THEM TO ADOPT POSITIVE THINKING HABITS

Encourage them to allocate time each day to practise all the procedures in the programme, including exercise and sensible eating. If possible, accompany them on their daily walk. You can talk at the same time.

We all embark on a new project with great enthusiasm, but after a couple of weeks the novelty starts to wear off as the discipline bites, and more seductive attractions present themselves. We start to question the value of what we are doing and are assailed by negative thoughts. This is the time for firm encouragement. Your depressed friend or partner will need to be continually reminded of the benefits that they, and incidentally you and your relationship, are deriving from the endeavour. Encouragement is needed, but be ready to be tough with them.

Listen, you and I have started this together and we are going to continue until you have completely tamed your Black Dog and put it back in its kennel. Got it? OK, let's get on with it. You mean too much to me to stop now.

Perseverance and continuity are the watchwords. The repair kit in this manual cannot rectify in a month or two the ravages of years of negative thinking. Nor can new ideas be imparted in so short a time. This manual is a day-to-day practical reference book for an enhanced and creative lifestyle. I hope that it will remain your companion long after the Black Dog has been banished. Helping involves participation and will enhance your life as well.

KNOW EACH OTHER'S METABOLIC CLOCKS AND CYCLES

Do not expect improvement like a straight-line graph. There will be periods of regression in taming the Black Dog and also in your relationship, especially if the depressed person is your spouse or partner. You too have a metabolic clock *(see Chapter 3)*. Both men and women have perfectly normal daily, weekly and monthly **low and slow times**, and these will inevitably interact with those of your partner. If you both find yourselves hitting a low at the same time, get out of each other's way. Give each other space. Go about your own business and follow your own inclinations. When you meet again you will both be refreshed.

John Gray, in his book *Men are from Mars, Women are from Venus*, proposes that in our relationships with each other men have a 'close and withdraw' mood tide roughly each month, whilst women experience an 'up and down' emotional wave each month. He uses this concept to help us to understand each other's needs and responses.

When women are on the downward part of their wave, he suggests, they need their man to be close and understanding. If the man is in his withdrawing mode at that time, there exists fertile ground for misunderstanding and disappointment with each other. Depression magnifies these quite normal emotional swings and roundabouts.

Whether you agree with Gray or not, the concept can be useful when you are helping someone in taming their Black Dog, Your metabolic clocks will affect the nature and spontaneity of your relationship, irrespective of whether you are partners, friends or colleagues, so be ready to disengage occasionally and to give each other plenty of fresh air.

DEPRESSION IN CHILDREN

It is reported that 40,000 school children are currently receiving medication for depression. This is represents a serious social problem, if parents do not understand that they, more than the doctor, have the key role to play in helping their child back to a positive and creative frame of mind. The other equally important person in a child's life at this time is their headteacher. Success in beating the Black Dog is dependent on the coordinated attention of parents and teacher with the support of the doctor. It is up to the parent and teacher working together in harmony to introduce focus, security, purpose and encouragement into the child's life.

Childhood is a fertile breeding time for inferiority complexes, and for acquiring unhealthy introspective feelings of being different to other children. Remember what the Jesuits are reported to have proclaimed: 'Give me a child until it is eight and you can do what you will with it after.' In short, at eight years old the indoctrination will be established in a child's mind – for the rest of his or her life. What enormous care we need to take, in nuturing these receptive little people!

What to look out for

Look again at the symptoms of depression on page x. The symptoms are the same with children but are more difficult to recognise because they may be suppressed. A child usually has not developed the skills to communicate how they are feeling. Indeed they may feel a sense of guilt about their feelings and conclude that they are just naturally lazy or incompetent. Here lies the foundation of a chronic inferiority complex because this is something they will not want to share with their parents or teachers. So recognising the presence of the Black Dog is an exercise in comparison.

Parents should watch out for pervading tiredness, lack of energy and a seeming reluctance to be involved in anything that needs concentration and resolution. Children usually love the excitement of trying out new things and testing adults to see how far they can go. If these healthy mischievous traits seem to be missing, cock your ears and twitch your muzzle.

Compare your child's performance and behaviour with that of other similar children. Compare changes in their own behaviour at different periods in their lives. Look out for a reluctance to compete – playing games is very important – and a tendency to capitulate in the face of difficulty or challenge.

Both parents should consider whether or not there are any manifestations of depression in their own lives. Was it a feature of your own childhood and has it recurred throughout your life, or are you affected at specific times of bereavement, major disruption and passing crises? Is there any evidence to suggest that your parents may have been afflicted?

The answers to these questions will indicate whether or not there is a family gene, which may give your child a propensity for depression. This information needs to be shared with your doctor, the child's teacher and the child him or herself, so that you all know the nature of the beast and can devise a plan for combating it.

Taming the Black Dog as a family

In a sense it is easier if one or both parents have suffered because you can adopt a family lifestyle for taming your Black Dogs. You can be open with each other regarding how you are feeling and hopefully your child will recognise that, rather like suffering from flu, depression is a condition that can be overcome. **Black Dogs are for taming**. Parent, teacher and child must learn to differentiate between the weariness of the affliction, which simply has to be addressed and overcome, and healthy tiredness from hard work or physical activity. They must eradicate negative thinking using the procedures in chapters 5, 6 and 7, and learn to recognise the elevating power of positive words.

> *Parents and teachers must understand that being attentive to a child's special needs is not to condone wayward behaviour. It is to take positive steps to help a young person to achieve their full creative potential.*

If your child's depression is not a family characteristic and is what I describe as a passing squall on life's sea, it still has to be taken very seriously. Passing squalls can catch you out and sink your vessel if you are not prepared to take appropriate action. The first step is to try to identify the underlying cause, because there is always an event or circumstance which triggers it off. Talk to your child, and more importantly, listen to what they have to say. Even if they seem not to want to talk to you about things, let them know that you are there when they need you. Your child's headteacher also needs to be consulted because your child spends more waking time in school than at home and is under constant observation there.

Causes of depression in school-age children

The causes of depression in a school-age child are many and varied and can be self-breeding. They can include bullying, parental pressure to do well in exams and tests, or being below par in physical pursuits, possibly resulting from a debilitating illness or surgery. Difficulties with school work are greatly magnified and will undermine a pupil's confidence so that they will find it difficult to ask their teacher for help.

Depression magnifies normal difficulties.

Bright and sensitive pupils can be handicapped by the influence of their less committed peers and can become depressed in the knowledge that in conforming to peer behaviour they are denying themselves the results they are capable of. Both parents and teachers need to be constantly vigilant for children becoming inhibited in this way. They must be ready to give support, encouragement and practical interest in helping them to handle this sort of pressure.

Resisting the sometimes demotivating effect of peer behaviour requires great strength of character and can lead to loneliness.

Throughout history it is the brightest, the gifted, the most talented and creative people who have proved to be most vulnerable to depression. It is therefore vital for a child's future that at the first suspicion of a Black Dog in your household you should consult your child's teachers. Do not wait for parents' day.

Obtain a meeting with the headteacher immediately and explain your suspicions. Ask for an evaluation of your child's potential. What are their best and worse subjects? Do they seem to have a special inclination for one particular subject and might it signify a latent talent worthy of special development? How quickly do they grasp what is being taught compared with other children and are their responses throughout a term consistent?

If at all possible both parents should attend the meeting with the head together. Go to listen and learn and ask the teachers for their advice in selecting something that the child can excel in. Encourage your child to take part in after-school clubs in whatever subject they are interested in: music, drama, sports, languages, chess, natural history, etc. If your school doesn't offer an appropriate club, look for other private groups, like a martial arts club or dance classes, for example – or alternatively, talk to the school about setting one up. This must not become an easy way out for a wayward child. They must participate in the full school curriculum in order for them to experience the enjoyment of success and the elevating feeling of achievement.

> *Success and achievement, accompanied by the admiration of parent, teacher and peer, will confound the Black Dog.*

Drugs and depression

There could well be a link between depression in young people and drug usage. Just as it is a cause of many adults becoming alcohol dependant, so some young people may well be seeking an escape from the weariness of depression with cocaine or cannabis and compensating for low self-esteem and diminished vitality with ecstasy and the like. I hasten to point out that I am not experienced in this field but it is a thought that parents, doctors and teachers alike need to bear in mind. It is easier for children under 16 to obtain drugs than it is for them to purchase alcoholic drinks.

The importance of sleep

Growing children need adequate sleep. However, getting the right amount of sleep is not about staying in bed in the morning, it is about going to bed at a proper time at night. In my opinion every child always has and always will require a full nine hours' sleep each night. Not nine hours in bed but nine hours of proper, healthy, refreshing, battery-charging sleep each night. This means being in bed by nine o'clock, with time for a bedtime story (read by you, or read themselves when they're older) and a cuddle before sleep.

We are all at our most vulnerable to a Black Dog attack at the time we open our eyes and start to contemplate the coming day. Children share this vulnerability. You must be able to differentiate between tiredness through lack of sleep on the one hand and the weariness brought about by the attentions of the Black Dog on the other. So, early to bed.

My silver-haired old Granny used to say, *'Every hour before midnight is worth two after. So pack up your Meccano set, there's a good boy, and off to bed. I'll come up to say goodnight in five minutes.'* Good old Granny. When she spoke we all had an uncharacteristic inclination to do as she bade. Today she might say that's the end of television tonight or it's computer closing time. The point I want to make is that Meccano packing-up time was precisely the same every night and everyone knew it. There was no argument. That was one of the rules of the household. Sleep is absolutely vital for health and to ensure that children get sufficient there have to be house rules that everyone conforms to, including mother and father.

Adequate sleep is vital for learning and for taming the Black Dog.

YOU CAN BENEFIT TOO

You do not need to be a depressive to benefit from this book. Many of the individual techniques that I recommend for taming the Black Dog have been utilised for generations by people seeking fulfilment in their lives. The difference here lies in the coordinated structure of the programme; the benefits accrue from the way the procedures focus on knocking out negative thinking with positive habits. You can use them equally well to improve the quality of your own life, as I have done.

Your own attitude of mind is crucial.

Keep a sense of proportion – both of you. Depression, like flu, is thoroughly unpleasant. Yes, it is debilitating. Yes, it is demoralising, but just like flu it comes and goes and is treatable. It is easy and rewarding to help someone with a sprained ankle or a broken collarbone or someone who has just undergone surgery, if only because invariably the patient is appreciative. The difficulty with helping someone with the Black Dog is that they are apt to transmit confused messages. Their body language can communicate aggressiveness, their demeanour is sullen and introspective and they tend to be uncommunicative. This may not reflect in any way the nature of their affection and respect for you, but because you cannot perceive a physical injury, it is difficult, at times impossible, for you to be compassionate. Don't worry. Stand back. Be detached. The squall will pass and normal service will be restored.

Try to hang on to your sense of humour – again both of you. There is always a funny side to everything if you look for it. It's an aspect of positive thinking. You should see my awakening antics when I am suffering. I have the undisputed record for getting from bed and to bath. I resemble, I am told, a cartoon cat being chased by an angry Black Dog. It's true.

SUMMARY

- Call it the Black Dog not depression.

- Persuade the sufferer to consult their doctor.

- Men will probably be stubborn and fearful while women may be shy and uncertain.

- Encourage them to establish responsive communications with the doctor and to change their GP if this proves impossible.

- Encourage discussion about the character and nature of the Black Dog.

- Depressives have a propensity for anger – if they become difficult, stand back.

- Encourage perseverance and praise progress with the programmes in this book.

- If you are concerned about your child, talk it through with them and with the headteacher and possibly your doctor.

- Know the timings of your own metabolic clock as well as theirs.

- Keep things in proportion.

- Try to maintain a sense of humour.

- Your task is to help a normal person to unload negative baggage and achieve their full potential.

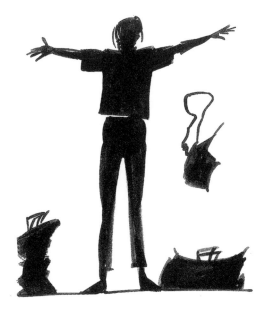

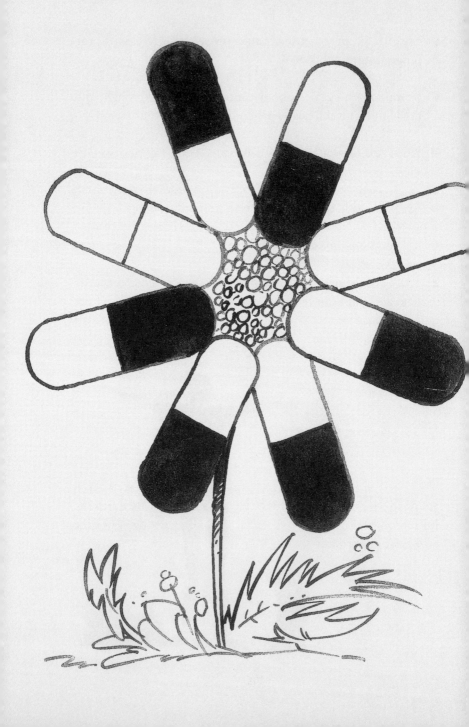

Appendix 1
Drug Treatments and Herbal Remedies

MEDICATION AND YOUR DOCTOR

Modern drugs are highly efficacious when properly prescribed, but mood-changing drugs by their very nature need to be continually monitored and this means establishing responsive communications with your GP.

Each drug has a highly focussed purpose and it is not unusual for there to be side effects of one sort or another. Side effects convey important messages to the doctor, so he or she must be informed regularly about feelings and reactions. When you have a good relationship with your doctor it is easy and perhaps understandable to overlook the fact that there are hundreds of patients with different levels of urgency demanding their attention as well as yourself. So the initiative must be with you to report on the efficaciousness of the medication on a regular basis.

This need not entail you losing one or two hours each week sitting in a surgery waiting room. By prior arrangement with the doctor, progress can be reported by telephone, saving your time and most importantly your doctor's time. The practice nurse in many cases is qualified to receive and pass on reports to the doctor.

I cannot over-emphasise the importance of establishing good communications with your GP. If you find it difficult or impossible to talk to him or her, then change to another. It is your right to do so.

DRUG TREATMENT

This is the exclusive province of your doctor and because I believe a little knowledge can be dangerous I have purposely refrained from including information about the different drug treatments. Suffice to say that each drug has a slightly different effect and some have significant side effects, which have to be weighed against the benefits.

The doctor's skill is to balance these factors with your physiology and your lifestyle, in order to select the most appropriate drug for your needs. Thereafter constant monitoring is necessary.

HERBAL REMEDIES

When considering trying out a herbal remedy, consult at least two experts before making a selection and consult with someone who is already using homeopathic solutions. Do not embark on such an experiment while you are taking medically prescribed drugs because they could interact detrimentally with each other. Consult your doctor before taking anything.

Disclaimer
All the following information is available in the public domain and is included purely in the interest of comprehensiveness. Unlike other parts of this book, the following information must not be construed as recommending a course of action.

St John's Wort

It is reported that in excess of 40 scientific studies have verified the effectiveness of this herb for the treatment of mild to moderate depression, it appearing to work in about 70% of cases. It commonly takes up to two weeks to have an effect, or a month in some cases. Tablets are usually taken with meals three times per day. Side effects, which have been reported, are mild stomach upset, rashes and restlessness.

Oats – *avena sativa*

The same oats from which you make porridge. They are reputed to be a very good tonic for the nervous system. The plant is used to combat anxiety, stress and fatigue as well as for depression. It is usually taken as a tea three times per day.

Lavender

Lavender has been traditionally used to promote relaxation and sleep in the form of a nosegay under a pillow. Its essential oil is available in most chemists and health food shops for applying to a pillow or for the bath.

Vervain – *verbena officinalis*

Traditionally used for the treatment of depression but not substantiated scientifically, it is said to have a nourishing and balancing effect on the whole nervous system. It is taken as a tea or as a tincture three times a day.

Kava-kava – *piper methysticum*

Alleviates the anxiety component of depression without sedation. Scientific studies of kava-kava indicate that it may improve memory and mental functioning.

Ginkgo - *ginkgo biloba*

Described as an amazing herb, it increases blood supply to the brain and improves nerve cell function. It enhances memory and intellectual activity and is reputed to be an excellent treatment for depression among the elderly. It is usually taken in capsule form three times per day.

Consult your herbalist before embarking on a course and talk to someone who has experience of using herbal treatments. Do not use them while taking prescribed drugs.

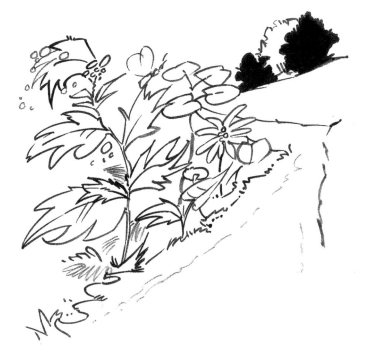

Useful organisations and contact details

Organisations able to provide immediate help or information concerning the Black Dog.

Patrick Ellverton
Website: www.Tamingtheblackdog.co.uk
Facilities include:
Residential courses
Personal counselling
Corporate courses

Herbalifestyle
Naunton
Cheltenham
Glos GL45 3AT
Tel: 01451 850341
Provides product information on nutritional vitality programmes.

Depression Alliance
35 Westminster Bridge Road
London SE1 7RJ
Tel: 0845 123 23 20
Email: information@depressionalliance.org
Website: www.depressionalliance.org
Depression Alliance is the leading UK charity providing information, support and understanding to anyone affected by depression. They provide a national network of self help groups, a variety of mutual support services and publications.

The Samaritans

Tel: 0857 909090 (24 hours)

A national 24-hour confidential, emotional support for anyone in crisis.

Saneline

Telephone helpline: 0845 767 8000

Tel: 020 7375 1002 (admin)

Email: sane@saneline.org

Website: www.saneline.org

Helpline offering emotional and crisis support to people experiencing mental illness, their carers, family and friends. Also provides information on mental health matters.

No Panic

Telephone helpline: 0808 808 0545 (10am to 10pm every day)

Tel: 01952 590 005 (admin)

Email: ceo@nopanic.org.uk

Website: www.nopanic.org.uk

No Panic offers a full range of services for people who suffer from panic attacks, phobias and obsessive/compulsive disorder.

Young Minds

102–108 Clerkenwell Road

London EC1M 5SA

Telephone helpline: 0800 018 1238

Tel: 020 7366 8445 (admin)

A service for parents and carers. The national children's mental health charity support scheme. Provides confidential information and advice for adults who are concerned with the mental health of a child or young person.

Parentline Plus
Telephone helpline: 0800 800 2222 (9am to 9pm Monday–Friday, 9.30 to 5pm Saturday, 10am to 3pm Sunday)
Fax: 020 7284 5501
Email: centraloffice@parentlineplus.org.uk
Website: www.parentlineplus.org.uk
Helpline and information for parents under stress.

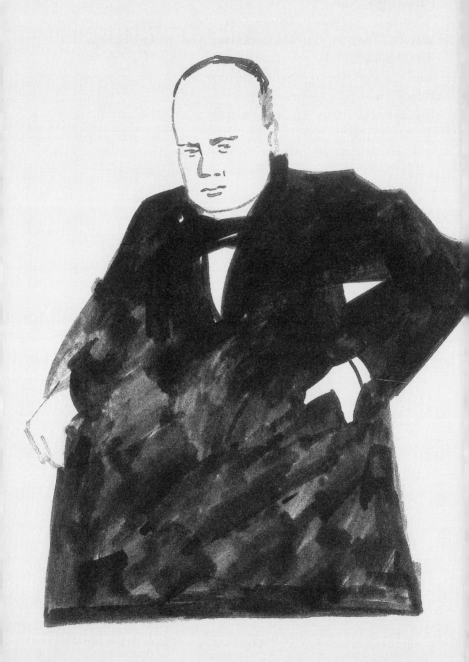

Appendix 3
Winston Churchill quotation – original version

Then turn again to your task. Look forward, do not look backward. Gather afresh in heart and spirit all the energies of your being, bend anew together for a supreme effort. The times are harsh, the need is dire, the agony of Europe is infinite, but the might of Britain hurled united into the conflict will be irresistible.

Index

If you want to know how...

- To buy a home in the sun, and let it out
- To move overseas, and work well with the people who live there
- To get the job you want, in the career you like
- To plan a wedding, and make the Best Man`s speech
- To build your own home, or manage a conversion
- To buy and sell houses, and make money from doing so
- To gain new skills and learning, at a later time in life
- To empower yourself, and improve your lifestyle
- To start your own business, and run it profitably
- To prepare for your retirement, and generate a pension
- To improve your English, or write a PhD
- To be a more effective manager, and a good communicator
- To write a book, and get it published

If you want to know how to do all these things and much, much more…

howtobooks

365 Steps to Self-Confidence

A programme for personal transformation in just a few minutes a day
David Lawrence Preston

Confidence is crucial to a happy and fulfilling life. It influences your success at work, your family life, relationships and leisure activities. It affects your performance in everything you do. A belief in one's self is without doubt the greatest asset of all. This book has been carefully structured to help you to achieve this crucial self-belief. It takes you deep inside your mind and gives you tools and techniques which have worked for millions of people around the world. All you have to do is work through and apply its lessons.

Time and energy devoted to building your confidence and self-esteem are nothing less than investments in your whole life.

"Dedicate time to read a chapter of this book every week and reap the benefits of growing more self-assured and confident...follow the 52 themed chapters, including exercises, insights and practical hints on how to overcome your lack of self-esteem and begin to live life to the full now, not tomorrow!" – Good Health

"I have spent pounds on books over the last few years but yours is worth a dozen of my collection." – Personal Development Trainer, Ireland

ISBN 978-1-84528-248-6

365 Ways to be Your Own Life Coach

A programme for personal and professional growth for just a few minutes a day
David Lawrence Preston

Life coaches aim to support and encourage their clients in their personal and professional growth by helping them to identify and achieve their goals. They use a variety of conversational and written techniques to help them find the best way forward, strengthen their motivation and take action. Good coaches don't give advice, but help the client to find the answer for themselves. But they are expensive.

If you follow the tried and tested methods offered in this book, you can transform your life with no financial outlay other than the cover price. The author bases his methods on three simple ideas:

■ The TGROW Method
■ Eight Steps to Success
■ The ITIA Formula

"I believe the best coach for you is you, and I aim to give free rein to that person. This book will show you exactly what you need to do to turn yourself into your own life coach. There are 365 priceless ideas, exercises and skills to learn from and apply. Finally, there is a 366th that will put all the rest in context."

ISBN 978-1-84528-058-1

Learning to Counsel

Develop the skills you need to counsel others
Jan Sutton and William Stewart

This practical book with its wealth of case studies, and examples of skills, illustrations and exercises, will be a valuable tool for anyone considering a career in counselling, for tutors of counselling skills courses and for many others who use counselling skills as a part of their work.

The framework of the book is based firmly in the person-centred approach of Carl Rogers and the skills-based approach of Gerard Egan. Counsellors can benefit from such models to guide them in their work. These, together with a repertoire of skills, and a careful study of the principles outlined here, will provide a basis for counselling practice. Indeed, it is our belief that the skills presented here can enhance all human relationships.

"…this excellent and user-friendly book is comprehensive and easy to read and comes alive with illustrative graphics and quotations. It is ideal for new and mature students in counselling and explains the core skills, conditions and model of counselling." – From the foreword by Neil Morrison, Director of the Institute of Counselling, Glasgow

"An inexpensive individual study resource which is aimed particularly at those studying to be counsellors." – Care and Health Magazine

"A counsellor's pocketbook and a useful companion to students on courses up to counselling skills certificate level." – Counselling and Psychotherapy Journal

ISBN 978-1-84528-325-4

Healing the Hurt Within

Understanding self-injury and self-harm and healing the emotional wounds
Jan Sutton

"This book is a giant leap forward in making self harm understandable to professionals and self-harmers alike." – Marjorie Orr, Director of Accuracy About Abuse

"Immensely readable and ultimately uplifting...has something to offer to anyone interested in understanding more about self-harming behaviour, whether at a personal or professional level." – Counselling at Work

"Aims to offer understanding, support and guidance... This is a book which will bring much comfort to the reader, be informative for family and friends, and can be used by practitioners to understand and work with those who self-harm." – Stress News

ISBN 978-1-84528-226-4

How To Books are available through all good bookshops, or you can order direct from us through Grantham Book Services.

Tel: +44 (0)1476 541080
Fax: +44 (0)1476 541061
Email: orders@gbs.tbs-ltd.co.uk
Or via our website: www.howtobooks.co.uk

To order via any of these methods please quote the title(s) of the book(s) and your credit card number together with its expiry date.

For further information about our books and catalogue, please contact:

How To Books
Spring Hill House
Spring Hill Road
Begbroke
Oxford
OX5 1RX

Visit our web site at
www.howtobooks.co.uk

Or you can contact us by email at info@howtobooks.co.uk